Praise for *Stepping Out* ...

I have often tried to find the right words to say to someone who is suffering, or to empathise with mental illness. Moving forward, I won't struggle because of this insightful story. I'll be giving a copy of *Stepping Out the Other Side: Finding Purpose Through Adversity* to anyone who asks me questions about mental illness in the future. We all have a role to play to make mental health a part of everyday conversation, and Pete inspired me to create a forum to do just that.

Chris Boyle, Founder of Poker Face
– Men's Mental Health

Pete Bell is someone I look up to personally and professionally. How Pete shares his story in *Stepping Out the Other Side: Finding Purpose Through Adversity* is real, raw and relatable. I believe all people, and especially people of influence, should read his story. I feel it will empower them to change the narrative around mental illness in the workplace. "The less people know, the better" will not serve the next generation.

Lachlan Stuart, Founder and Director of
The Man That Can Project

Stepping Out the Other Side: Finding Purpose Through Adversity is a moving story. It is full of wisdom and is very life affirming, intelligent and well written. It provides readers with a positive and relatable approach to move forward post adversity.

Richard Roberts, Founder and Director of
Suicide Prevention Pathways

Peter Bell's written work is a true and authentic demonstration of the challenges experienced from within. It is a cautionary reflection of the damage we can inadvertently do to ourselves, and by extension the people around us, when we lower our guard and stray from our values. His story personifies the challenges associated with fighting the destructive voice within one's own head and conveying the importance of connection to our purpose and our loved ones. *Stepping Out the Other Side: Finding Purpose Through Adversity* is a must read for those people who are feeling lost and require guidance by example.

David Neal, Co-Founder and Director of The Eighth Mile Consulting

These days in mental health care to draw on 'lived experience' is an essential pillar of everything that we do, from designing services, to conducting research and to advocating for reform of and investment in our much-neglected mental health 'system'.

Unlike with other health areas, some of the lived-experience narrative is hostile to health professionals and medical researchers and undermines our efforts. Such hostility, driven as it is by the neglect and poor-quality care of the mentally ill over the decades, is understandable but needs to be channelled better and balanced by hope and strategy.

So, it is very refreshing to read Pete Bell's inspirational story. *Stepping Out the Other Side: Finding Purpose Through Adversity* describes the value of expert clinical care which, combined with his own personal coping strength, invaluable family support and a strong philosophical base, enabled him to win his battle against mental illness.

It is also refreshing to hear the threat of mental illness described in this way as a fight or a battle which implies that victory, or at least resistance, is possible. Contrast this with what is typically said: that people 'battle' cancer but 'suffer' from mental illness. The analogy with heavy-weight boxing is evocative.

Pete also makes the crucial distinction between mental health and mental illness which so many of us fail to grasp. He points out:

In my opinion, mental illness and mental health are two separate concepts. Everybody has to make wise and conscious choices to manage their own mental health. There is an element of self-control and personal responsibility in influencing one's own mental health. In contrast, exceptional mental health man-agement won't always avert a mental illness. The illness can develop beyond a person's control, desire and avoidance effort.

This distinction is very timely as we navigate the threat of the coronavirus pandemic. It confirms that 'resilience' is not a protector from mental illness. Indeed, most people who have to fight mental illness display more resilience in doing so than the average person ever does. Resilience is a consequence not a barrier against stress or crisis. Pete is a wonderful example of and role model for this.

I believe Pete's story gives a voice to the wide main-stream of people in Australia who experience mental ill-health and mental illness. He shares a constructive way forward for all of us, the 5 million Australians each year, rising to more than 50% of us over time, with 'lived experience', the doctors and other health professionals, the medical researchers and the policy makers, to fight for a fair deal for the mentally ill.

Professor Patrick McGorry AO,
Professor of Youth Mental Health (Uni of Melbourne),
Executive Director of Orygen,
Founding Director of Headspace

STEPPING OUT THE OTHER SIDE

Finding Purpose Through Adversity

Peter Bell

Published in Australia in 2020 by Peter Bell

Email: peter@aurelius.com.au
Website: www.aurelius.com.au

ISBN 9780648871705 (paperback)

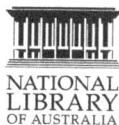

A catalogue record for this book is available from the National Library of Australia

Disclaimer

The information contained in this book is not intended to be a substitute for medical advice and professional health support under any circumstances. It is for general purposes only. Please seek help from a health professional immediately if you have any concerns regarding your mental wellbeing.

To my wife and little girl – my everything
To Mum and Dad, for everything

Contents

Foreword

I first met Pete Bell at a cafe in my local town of Mooloolaba, Queensland. A few weeks prior, Pete had emailed me and introduced himself as a fellow coach and philosophical enthusiast, and he wondered if we might meet for a chat one day when he had planned to be in my area. Having recently left my job to pursue a more meaningful path, I was optimistic about what might be a mutually beneficial meeting of two like-minded professionals.

The Roman statesman and playwright, Seneca, once wrote to his friend Lucilius, "Certainly you should discuss everything with a friend; but before you do so, discuss in your mind the man himself. After friendship is formed you must trust, but before that you must judge." Despite what might seem like a hyper-social outer shell, I'm usually quite reluctant to give my friendship quickly when I meet a new person. When I met Pete, however, the process of judgement and the feeling of trust were one and the same. From the moment I sat down with him, I felt a strong sense that this was a person who I could discuss anything with. His calm, humble and mild-mannered presence was immediately reassuring and, in a world of posturing and synthetic appearances, Pete showed me what it truly means to embody authenticity and mindfulness. This was not a meeting of two professionals, but rather it was the immediate uniting of two friends.

Within only a brief moment, we had finished with the pleasantries and were now going straight into the good stuff – the kind of conversation that makes life worth living. We discussed books, philosophy, mental health, coaching, and everything in between. Neither I nor Pete held anything back and, before we knew it, we had spent an hour and a half together – with not a second wasted.

I know that what I found in Pete that day you, too, will find in this book. You'll meet a person who has learned what it means to live with true self-awareness, gratitude, and personal responsibility. And above all, I know that you'll find a friend – someone who is willing to open their life to you in a hope that you might find some common ground and some personal understanding through the lens of their experience.

Mental (brain) health complications are at pandemic levels in the world today and, despite the efforts of many wonderful people and organisations, we still have a long way to go on the journey to better understanding, diagnosis and treatment. I can remember the way that I perceived mental health when I was younger, and I'm not proud to say that my perceptions were misinformed to say the least. Many people still believe, as I once did, that overcoming mental health issues is a game of 'mind over matter'. Unfortunately, this kind of thinking too often leads those suffering from poor mental health to feel isolated and helpless in their struggle. This book offers an inside look into the mind of someone who has not only endured a mental illness, but who has also learned to integrate this disorder into his life in a way that has vastly improved his wellbeing and that of his family and his community. It is a hero's journey of epic proportions, and one which is to be admired, learned from, and replicated.

Pete is a unique person in today's world. He tells the truth, speaks honestly about his strengths and weaknesses, and genuinely desires to only aim at the good. This, in my opinion, makes him a diamond in the rough. Read on to see why.

Simon J Drew

Author's Note

If only one piece of vital information exists within this book, please let it be that appropriate help is sought immediately for any personal suffering. This is a courageous act. Do not tell yourself anything else.

If previous attempts to find help did not deliver the required outcomes. Please don't let this be a barrier to trying again. Don't give up. Keep searching for a different perspective – a new way of looking at the specific set of circumstances. I am living proof this is worth it.

Throughout this story, the words 'mental illness' will consistently appear. When these words do appear, I encourage you to visualise one of the largest organs in the human body; this is the brain.

Like any physical component of the human body, the brain can also break. It may not be under exactly the same circumstances as an arm or a leg. There is a similar lack of control associated with such an unfortunate and painful occurrence.

I am yet to meet a person who would choose the pain and hardship associated with a broken bone. Mental (brain) illness deserves the same context. Everyone is susceptible to broken bones. Everyone is also susceptible to mental illness. It does not no discriminate.

My personal experience is that some people find it difficult to engage around mental illness. Humans fear what they do not understand. Given one cannot feel or see mental (brain) illness, it is a confronting topic for many. This uncertainty magnifies in people who have not experienced such challenges firsthand.

Time, wisdom and greater empathy have all provided me with a more balanced perspective on the situation. I now appreciate that this lack of engagement is not always because people don't care. They often don't know how to approach the situation in a confident manner.

This story exists to offer hope – hope to keep fighting and moving forward, especially when no visible path exists. The story is not only for people who battle through mental illness. We all share one irrefutable commonality: we are all human beings, relatable on so many more levels than we often acknowledge.

Given this story is for everyone, I have deliberately chosen a clear, concise and direct communication style. Anyone who wishes to do so should be able to read this story. Ironically, this style also reflects the balance and simplicity I now require in my life. Mental illness is already a complex topic. It won't help advance people's understanding by complicating it further, nor will romanticising it improve the situation.

Throughout history, a number of wise individuals have insinuated that writing a short letter takes up too much time, so just write a long one instead. This wisdom is not lost on me. Hence, this is a relatively short story.

Please don't link the length of the story to the intensity of the fight. Such battles actually don't have time stamps. They require a never-ending focus and continual support. My fight is not over; it is continual.

My story is important if it can help others. I do not feel that it is special or unique. It is surprisingly common in society. Everyday people are not sharing enough of these stories and they need to become normalised.

Lifeline reports that suicide remains the leading cause of death in Australia for people aged 15 to 44. The challenge around this national health crisis is immense. I finished high school in 1997. Sadly, five men from my grade have taken their own life since then. I kept these five men and their families deep in my thoughts while writing this story.

So why is suicide still referred to as the silent killer? This has to change.

Everyone is responsible and has a critical role to play in facilitating this change. Greater levels of encouragement around honest, transparent and empathetic dialogue must occur. This is a tragic situation. I for one feel like I no longer have a choice. Enough is enough and I must speak and share my experience.

I am blessed that I have an encouraging support network around me. I find myself in a very fortunate position where I can take time to share this story.

Many other people do not have this same level of support. This is not lost on me. My words will never do justice to what some must endure alone. These people are the overlooked and understated warriors of our world. They deserve a louder voice.

I felt it was also important to pay respect to those who kindly support others with mental illness. It takes an equal amount of patience, courage and tenacity. I have witnessed this challenge with my family and close friends who all support me unconditionally. I wouldn't be where I am today without them.

Thank you for giving up your precious time and allowing me to share my story with you.

Pete Bell
May 2020

Prologue

Owning our story can be hard; but not nearly as difficult as spending our lives running from it.
— *Brené Brown*

Irreversible damage across all facets of my life was now afoot. Hopelessness cascaded across my entire body. Head to toe, I felt heavy and poisoned with dread. Every conceivable thought told me I couldn't recover from this.

Wednesday 27 February 2019 was the second evening of my hospital stay. Reality set in that everything I had known about my life was now broken. My relationships, friendships, career and my own soul were all in a pure state of chaos.

For the first time in my life, I was shit scared. It felt like heavy chains were locking me to the bed – not physical chains, mental ones that were pulled so tight I could no longer move. I was paralysed with fear and trapped, a prisoner inside my own head.

I was becoming desperate. If an out existed, I wanted it. Other people must have been in this unfortunate position before. How the hell did they find comfort and start to loosen the tight grips of insanity?

I needed relief. I needed inspiration. I needed a relatable story.

What type of person would write such a story?

An everyday person who has messed up and applied one too many bandaid fixes. A person pulled closer to the edge of a tall building by some force of nature far stronger and powerful than their own will. A petrified person, perilously having their subconscious take more ground in the battle. A person that managed to outsmart the den of deluded beasts in their head. One that lived to tell the tale and step out the other side.

I need this story. It may be my last hope.

Someone, please help me.

SHIT …

Inner Turmoil

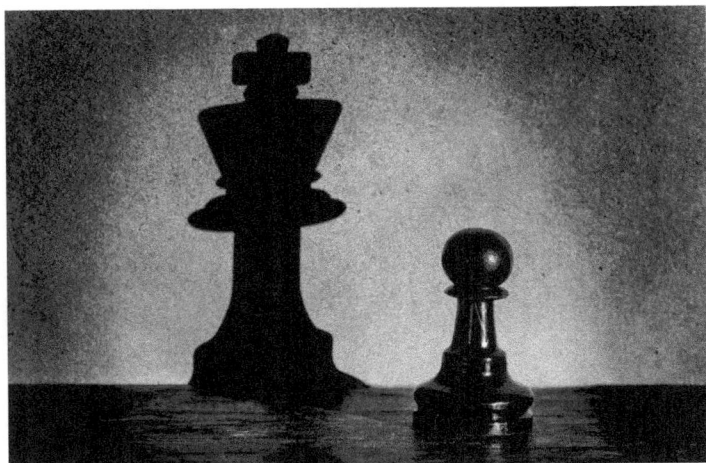

Things are not always what they seem; the first appearance deceives many; the intelligence of a few perceives what has been carefully hidden.

— Phaedrus

On Tuesday 26 February 2019, I became a patient at a private hospital. It was a surprisingly pleasant facility. Care existed for people with a variety of medical conditions, including substance addictions, mental illness and postnatal depression.

People from the local neighbourhood would not be out of place. Even close friends or relatives could find themselves walking these corridors. Everyday people were everywhere – people like me, who had denied the extent of their internal challenges for too long. People that now needed saving from themselves.

My hospitalisation was a sudden, unplanned medical intervention. I deliriously believed it would be a short two-day stint. I had no need to get too comfortable with any hospital schedule or visit the communal dining room.

I would be back at work in no time, doing the one thing that I loved most. Fingers crossed I didn't succumb to the strong urges: the urges to plough my car head-first into a pole or any other fixed concrete object on the way. I was pretty confident I would make it there. My work colleagues needed me. No way would I ever let them down.

I was blissfully unaware of the dark clouds compounding on the stormy horizon. Unbeknown to myself, I was extremely unwell. I had been living a lie to everyone around me, including myself. I had been avoiding my scariest reality of all: facing my mental illness head on.

This was all about to change. A ten-minute meeting with my new psychiatrist was all it took. He searched my bag and removed anything sharp. He confiscated two coat hangers. My tried and tested tactic of bullshitting wasn't working. He saw right through it. This was not his first rodeo.

There was no grey area left post meeting. He was not joking around. This would be a minimum one-and-a-half-week stay. It could be much longer. The majority of people stay an average of two months. He observed that these people also have beautiful families like mine. It made me feel like the least I could do was commit to one-and-a-half weeks for my young family.

The welcome to my come-to-Jesus moment had taken place. My existential crisis: a state of inner turmoil that had been 38 years in the making.

Twenty-four hours is not a long time. In the context of my hospitalisation, it felt like a lifetime. I cracked and reality rapidly set in. There was no false bravado left. I was a defeated man.

The following section represents a snapshot of my journal entries and thoughts. I wrote these during my hospital stay, often outside in the fresh air. This is where

I felt some normality and peace – an escape from the four walls inside.

These entries helped me make sense of something that was so foreign and to start my long journey of healing. It was a comforting behaviour for an uncomfortable situation.

These journal entries are unstructured and raw to better reflect the reality of my hospitalisation.

Denial – Wednesday 27 February 2019

I still can't believe I find myself in this position.

Deep down I will need every bit of courage to see this through. I am shameful and shit scared. My family doesn't deserve to suffer any longer.

Anxiety follows me everywhere; it's rampant. It sends me into such an unhealthy place. I snap at the little things. I am distant; I am irritable. I become an asshole. I don't want to be an asshole any longer, especially not to those I love the most.

I am scared I can't fix this.

I am scared of the consequences of my family losing me.

I am scared of my beautiful daughter growing up without a dad or my supportive wife without a husband. They deserve far better in life.

I hope coming here will finally give me a circuit breaker. I need to change some things in my life for the better. I need to adjust my expectations of myself. This self-hate can't continue any longer.

I can't try and beat the world anymore. It is too big. Others may have conquered it but that won't be me.

I have battled this now for 38 years and know it will never end or leave me. It is a part of the person I am.

Success to me was to never break down and end up in a hospital broken. Now here I am. What an absolute failure.

I have given everything to try to manage this myself. I have proven I can't do it.

I am a prisoner trapped in my own head as my emotions keep shifting: one minute, courageous, the next, I am shameful.

Having my three-year-old daughter and wife check me into hospital because I am broken makes my heart ache. Or will my daughter grow up better for knowing it's courageous to ask for help? Will she even see me as a role model? Not some shameful, mentally broken failure.

And what do those two girls deserve? Nothing but the best.

To have fought so hard to get our beautiful little girl … She is a real angel and, to think, I may have jeopardised our family unit? What an absolute fool.

Alone with your own thoughts at night in this hospital is a frightening situation.

You question many things:
- Who have I let down?
- What will people think of me?

- Will people look at me as a failure?
- How will I ever work again?
- How will I support my family?

The rumination continues. I don't know how this can end well.

Sorrow – Thursday 28 February 2019

Nurses kept checking on the man in bed next to me all night, every hour. Poor guy might be on suicide watch.

Despite how dark things are, I get up and do the only thing I know that will be beneficial. I start walking around the inside perimeter of the hospital.

I am sad today. I am trying to be as brave as possible, but the reality is still hitting me of where I am and why I am here.

Tears stream down my face as I catch a glimpse of myself in the cafe window.

Is that me? How did I let this happen?

I am a total stranger trapped in my own head, wanting to get out and be the real me, the best version of me.

What a joke. I can't even work out how I am going to get a towel for my shower in this place. How can I even think about the best version of myself?

My shame and embarrassment have magnified. The thought of how many people this impacts in a negative way crosses my mind.

My wife has had to tell her work; my work colleagues suffer. My parents will stress. They will feel hopeless that they can't help.

I am now sitting at the coffee shop alone, balling my eyes out.

I have a thought of walking down to the intersection at the main road and looking at the cars, just to see what it feels like. Would I run out in front of one?

That's not what I want. My family needs me here but, at this point, I am as low as I can get.

The guilt, shame and embarrassment are next level.

What a useless idiot. How did you not see this coming and avoid it? So much for your intelligence.

Now all these people suffer because of your incapability to manage your own shit.

I begin to look at photos of my two beautiful girls. I need to ground myself back into the reality of what's important.

Perspective – Friday 1 March 2019

My wife and little girl insisted on coming to visit me. A part of me wants to shelter them from this journey. I don't want them to see me this broken.

They say it will make them happy. The thought that I could make someone happy at the moment is baffling.

I sit in the waiting room for at least an hour waiting for their arrival. I have never wanted to see people so much in all my life.

I watch every car drive up the hill, waiting and hoping for it to be the girls.

My beautiful wife would be under so much pressure at the moment. She is now working almost full-time, plus looking after our little girl, managing the family affairs, and dealing with my shit.

The admiration I have for her cannot be expressed with mere words. She is a rock and I love her dearly. Her commitment to me is unconditional.

The simple takeaway meal I share with the girls at the hospital is one I will never forget. Everything about it reminded me of what is important in life.

On the way out, I purchased a bag of lollies from the vending machine for my little girl. It made her so happy; her reaction melted my heart.

I went to bed in a much calmer state tonight. All thanks to the girls.

Reflection – Monday 4 March 2019

I met with my psychiatrist and it helped. He is smart and already understands me. He has provided some strategies to help. This includes changing my dosage of medication.

I spent considerable time working on exercises for the psychiatrist. One was to track my entire life history, noting major milestones and mental health challenges.

At the end of the exercise, we identified that I have had five breakdowns in my life. The first was at the age of nine or ten, while in grade five. The fifth is my current situation.

What do I mean by breakdown? It has changed for me over the years, but my mind breaks and can no longer function.

Initially, rational and logical thoughts flood my mind, like solving work problems.

The challenge arises when it gets overloaded. When it gets pushed too far with rational thoughts, it malfunctions and irrational thoughts take over.

My mind perceives these irrational thoughts as real. I can no longer think straight. I can't define what is real or false.

I want to escape. I want to kill my broken mind.

Killing my physical body to silence my mind remains a scary thought. I don't want this. It is something of which I am fearful.

Why do I keep pushing my mind to this point of breaking?

I sense it may be some form of deep insecurity and lack of self-confidence. I am always trying to reach a point of achievement. A target that enables me to value and appreciate myself.

It feels like a form of addiction. I need to break this repetitive cycle. That is why hospital is the best place for me at the moment. I can't be trusted to do this alone.

To provide perspective, the work office closed for the end-of-year break on the Wednesday before Christmas. This concluded the most intense year of my working career.

Thursday night, I spent eight hours getting an online accreditation in coaching.

Friday, I went into the office to print out lecture notes. I needed these notes for a coaching diploma I would complete during our family holiday.

I spent Saturday getting another online accreditation. I wanted to learn psychometric testing skills. This took me five hours.

By Sunday, I had signed up to complete more coaching accreditations over the break. I had also started working towards completing them.

Monday was Christmas Day. While I loved the day with family, deep down I would have liked to be somewhere else. I wanted more time to progress my achievements.

I consciously knew that what I was doing was selfish, but I couldn't stop. Demons possess others, and I felt possessed.

I had managed to convince myself that it would be different this time. I could handle all this now. I was more self-aware.

I would get inside my own head and tell myself that I was a useless piece of shit. This would motivate me. I needed to get all this done now or I was as weak as piss.

Caring work colleagues or family members would sometimes ask if I was ok. I would smile and say everything was great. The scary thought is that, at this stage, I thought everything was great myself. Similarly, if people tried to call me out on lying, I would flip my lid and get angry. These poor people couldn't win with me.

It doesn't register at all that I am courageous. Breaking down five times now and fighting back is no easy task, I guess. I think I am messed up. I still think courageous people are the ones that can achieve so much but never end up with broken minds. They are the mentally tough ones that I admire.

Is it a form of courage to keep pushing myself to the brink and not settle for mediocrity? It results in growth, but this growth comes at a cost. This cost now spreads far wider than me. I have a responsibility to an amazing family.

15

I see that it was selfish behaviour now that I am reflecting on things. In many ways, it was not the real me. I hope it wasn't, anyway.

Family – Tuesday 5 March 2019

I had my first group session on Cognitive Behavioural Therapy and I met some great people.

There are many misconceptions about what this type of hospital is like, especially in relation to the types of people here. I have met many wonderful, kind-hearted people already.

My mum also came to visit me today in hospital. I was a little apprehensive about this visit initially. Like the girls, I don't want Mum and Dad feeling any extra burden from this mess I have created.

She was also not aware of the decision made for me to come to hospital until after the fact.

My brother still doesn't know I am here. This signifies the speed at which everything happened. I guess this is a brutal reminder of how quickly things deteriorated for me.

I am well aware that this would be a tough situation for any parent to find themselves in with their children. In the end, I figured, like any caring parent, she would likely stress more if she didn't get to visit me.

It was definitely the right decision; Mum and I had a great chat for around two hours. It was a very practical conversation around the complexities of my mental health.

We even had a few laughs about the scars I have ended up with along the journey. Mum was very understanding and supportive as always.

Mum also told me she was very proud of me. Despite having my challenges, I had always pushed myself and had a crack at everything.

I could have easily felt sorry for myself and played the victim. This is the last outcome I ever wanted in my life. To hear Mum say she was proud meant the world to me. It provided some relief to my compromised state of mind.

Oblivious – Thursday 7 March 2019

I decided this morning to walk up the large hill that forms the hospital entrance as many times as possible. I got to a total of five when it started to pour down with rain and I had to stop. I am bitterly disappointed with this lack of achievement.

I caught up with my psychiatrist this morning. I was wearing an old Nirvana shirt – interesting choice considering the current situation.

Given my perceived interest in music, he asked me if I had ever seen a documentary about Quincy Jones?

He casually mentioned that Quincy and I share some similarities. We are both pig-headed and extremely driven pricks.

I said thank you with pride. I felt pretty chuffed with this compliment.

The psychiatrist also told me that most people can only walk the hill six times. I told him immediately that I would finish the hill over ten times within the next few days. He just politely smiled back at me.

My psychiatrist is excellent and I really like him. His assessment and work with me to date has been eye-opening.

He takes the time to consider different perspectives, asking me questions to better understand my mind – questions I now wish other doctors had asked me previously.

I am guessing I have some form of a compulsive personality disorder. I take things to the deepest and most intense point possible, most likely to avoid some form of anxiety, guilt or shame, maybe?

I don't fully know as yet. That's why he is the psychiatrist; he will work it out.

I did the hill eleven times this afternoon.

I will see what the psychiatrist has to say next time I see him. I'm pretty sure he won't be overly surprised.

I could have done more. My calf muscles did start to ache, but that's just an excuse. I also don't want my psychiatrist to think I am too much of a psycho.

Stigma – Saturday 9 March 2019

I took hospital leave and went and watched ballet this morning. I really enjoyed it.

My little girl was so focused and attentive to her teachers. She is beautiful.

I came back to the hospital after my half-day visit outside. I felt like I needed to come back. I miss the girls like crazy but feel I am not ready for the wider world.

This is going to take time if executed properly. I am now warming to this plan.

The psychiatrist has doubled the dosage of my current medication. This seems 100% the right thing to do. However, it makes me more anxious and quite nauseous in the initial stages, until I adjust to the side effects.

It might be the medication, but this afternoon I am questioning what my life will look like on the outside. It can't be the same future as before I arrived here.

I know I am a fighter; I have proven this for 38 years. I know how to get back up when I get knocked down. But I also know I have a tendency to chase the initial punch in the face.

This will be a different challenge for me. How am I going to slow down and live a life that is not full of pushing myself every day?

Deep down, I know a slower life is right for the girls. Therefore, it must also become right for me.

But this will be foreign. And the fear of the unknown always manifests as something far worse in your mind than in reality.

I am also starting to dread having to explain myself on the outside. Facing the stigma associated with mental illness is not going to be a pleasant task.

I am amazingly supported by those who matter most to me. However, I still feel that many in society judge on this front. Perhaps, it is all in my head.

Having to explain myself to others, who may insinuate that I am weak, is a shit situation. Any comment that I came to hospital to avoid other circumstances will cut me deep. This will feel like a knife being lodged in my heart.

I am not in the blame game, and I am grateful for everything I have, even for my mental illness. It makes me the person I am.

Sometimes, I can become a lost / anxious / guilty / frustrated / low / worrisome / negative / angry / over-thinking / obsessed / compulsive / distant / lacking-self-confidence person. And the different versions of this person can come and go like the wind.

But I am never an untrustworthy / dishonest / ungrateful / judgemental / arrogant or entitled person. And maybe, I have my mental illness to thank for these admirable character traits.

I hope people afford me a level of respect that fairly reflects my character – character that has been built over the past 38 years.

Being in hospital is not my deliberate choice. I am a functioning person with a high level of responsibility in life. Why would I put myself through the guilt, shame, hurt and embarrassment if I wasn't broken?

I needed help.

Sense – Sunday 10 March 2019

I am leaving hospital for good later today. I am departing somewhat relieved but equally apprehensive. Life on the outside will be a delicate balancing act.

It is starting to make more sense why I was here, especially when I examine my life's history in greater detail.

My belief of never being good enough has driven huge feelings of anxiety and guilt. Obsessive thoughts must flow from this core belief system. Compulsive behaviours manifest to calm everything down.

For instance, I must work, learn or grow until breaking. I need these compulsive behaviours, otherwise I sense extreme guilt and anxiety. If I don't achieve at this level, I let others down.

It all reinforces the fundamental belief system that I am never good enough. This becomes a dangerous, self-repeating feedback loop in my brain.

When I was younger, I used to wash my hands consistently as a compulsive behaviour. Washing my hands would ease the uncomfortable anxiety. This anxiety flowed from the obsessive thought of having contracted a life-threatening disease.

It would appear that the compulsive behaviours can change over time. The obsessive thoughts can also change over time. Unfortunately, the pattern never changes.

The pattern remains firm. The reason being that the fundamental belief system doesn't change. The belief that I am never good enough reflects an immoveable object.

If someone tries to stop these compulsive behaviours, I am quick to anger. They are taking away my coping mechanism, making me sit with the uncomfortable feelings of guilt or anxiety.

Mental illness is complex, especially for people who have never walked the path themselves. For instance, I was always diagnosed with general anxiety and depression.

I am now aware that obsessive-compulsive disorder is my underlying mental illness. Depression can be a potential flow on effect, but it is not the condition that needs treatment.

The root cause of my challenges was unknown. Hence, it wasn't managed effectively.

The obvious example is the difference in appropriate levels of medication required. Obsessive-compulsive disorder required a 100% increase in my medication level – double the dosage prescribed to me for general anxiety or depression. My brain requires extra levels of serotonin to function.

The ability for my psychiatrist to take the time and dig deeper has made a huge difference. He has gotten to the root cause of the real problem.

It has been a long time coming, this accurate diagnosis. It's something that no one else has taken the time to do over the years. This is a huge relief.

I am so grateful to my general practitioner doctor and this hospital. I am scared of where I may have ended up and what may have happened if this intervention didn't take place.

The general practitioner doctor could see how broken my mind was that first day in her surgery. She knew hospital was the only place for me and she was right.

Deep Work

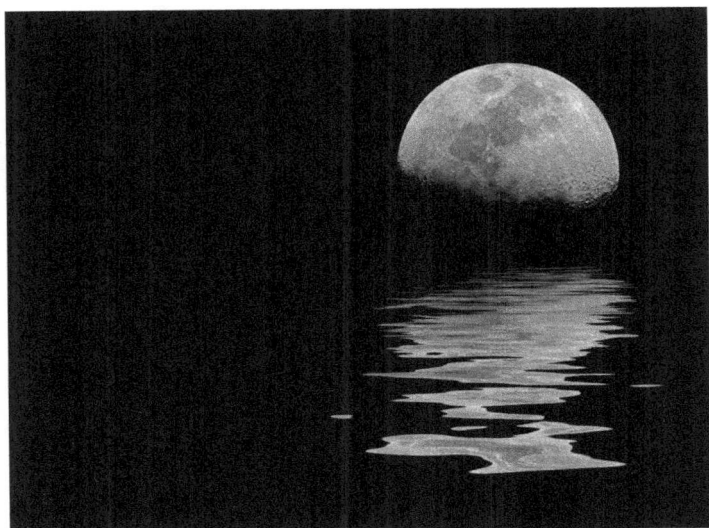

All the beauty of life is made up of light and shadow.
— Leo Tolstoy

I stared out the passenger seat window of my father-in-law's car as it pulled slowly into our driveway. The girls couldn't pick me up from hospital due to important family commitments. Nevertheless, it was comforting to see the familiar sight of home again. Everything was still as it seemed. The lawn did appear longer than when I departed. This shouldn't be a problem; I now had ample time to mow. I suspected many home duties would be on my new agenda. Something always needed fixing around the home. I did wonder where my own mind should rank on this fix-it list for life back on the outside.

Our little dog ran to greet me, jumping up with pure excitement. It was like her best friend had returned from a long overseas holiday. There is something beautiful about the non-judgemental and unconditional love of a dog. She wouldn't differentiate between my invisible mental illness and a visible physical injury. This differentiation is much harder for humans to make, especially for me.

Spending time in hospital isn't always pleasant. There are obviously different levels to the resultant pain and suffering. The return home is often a joyous occasion, surrounded by get-well-soon cards, balloons hanging from the ceiling and flowers blooming in vases. Well-wishers are eager to drop in and pass on their regards.

On Sunday 10 March 2019, after I was released from hospital, I returned to none of this. It was delusional and naive to think I would. My nearest and dearest were of course relieved to see me back home. However, counting the people who knew of my hospitalisation was a simple task. I could achieve this on my right-hand fingers. My brother and best friends were still not aware.

I'd made this decision. I was commander and chief in charge. I wouldn't budge. The less people that knew, the better. I could not handle the thought of anyone knowing. This scared the shit out of me. My ultimate moment of weakness on public display for full judgement? No thanks.

My internal courage was lacking. I was about to learn the hard way that this needed to change. I thought I was relatively self-aware. In reality, I knew so little about a deeper part of myself: the subconscious that controls around 95% of thoughts, behaviour and patterns. Hospital was challenging, but the hardest fight was yet to come. Shit was just getting real.

* * *

I was back in the real world. Everyone was living their life and dealing with their own challenges. I had created this reality for myself. As much as I needed wider support, I was not prepared to risk my pride for such a privilege. I had made the bed, and now it was time to lie in it.

I was still broken, and I no longer had the shelter from reality that hospital had so generously provided. My wife was working. My parents, and in-laws, would check in with me daily. I would always reply that I was doing fine and making progress when they worriedly enquired. I was quickly back to my old tricks again in that regard.

I did not know if, or when, I would ever be able to work again. We had vast insurance cover in place as a family. Disappointingly, this would not provide any financial benefit, given a pre-existing condition clause. My work kindly offered to support me financially for a period of time. This could not be a long-term viable solution. It was already clear that a return to my previous role was not a wise option.

I was also dealing with a significant case of lost identity. One minute, I was performing my profession at the highest level for a successful organisation. Next, I was staring down the barrel of not being mentally fit to do any paid job.

I was a proud person. My belief system was strong and unwavering. I perceived my career as the only thing in which I was ever successful at in life. This was deeply ingrained in my psyche. My work was my identity; it was what gave me my purpose. Under no circumstances would I ever want this taken from me.

But it was now lost. At least from my perspective anyway. It was like ripping the most sizeable chunk out from my heart. One day while brushing my teeth, I caught a glimpse of myself in the mirror. The person looking back was a stranger. Not even 10% of the person I once believed myself to be.

This first week outside of hospital and back in the real world was dangerous. It was like living on a knife edge.

I could only function for a very small period of time. I could concentrate for a five-minute phone conversation or face-to-face discussion. I could quickly get a takeaway coffee from the local cafe. I could not process anything greater.

My mind was still full – filled with guilt, shame, sadness and other negative ruminations. There was little space for anything else. Externally, I was a zombie – a zombie trying to make it through five-minute intervals of time, my mind so damaged and dislocated from reality that each five-minute interval felt like five hours.

On Wednesday 13 March 2019, I sat on our family couch alone in silence. I simply stared at the ceiling. My wife came home to check on me before going to pick our little girl up from day care. In a caring manner, she asked what I had done during the day. I just looked at her blankly. I struggled to find the appropriate words, especially given all I had achieved that day was to stare at the ceiling and sleep for an extended period of time.

The conversation concluded with my wife asking me for a small favour. I knew it was more than a favour. It was polite encouragement to help move me forward. My poor wife was most likely looking for a sign of hope. Hope she could get her husband back, the man she had married – the calm, considered, capable and balanced human I'd once been.

The request was simple enough. I was to pick up some grocery items from the local store for her, a ten-minute exercise at most.

* * *

The next day, I went to the shop. I regrettably never took shopping bags. This was a classic representation of my flawed belief system. I will sort it out myself. I didn't need any help. That would be a sign of weakness. I couldn't let anyone see that, especially not myself.

It was a challenge but I managed to get the items into the car. I dumped them on the back seat. They rolled around everywhere during the short drive home. Upon reaching home, I found that my wife and little girl had arrived about one minute before me. They were in the driveway waving as I pulled up.

This would be a proud moment. I could show my wife that I was ready to move forward. I had delivered on her request. I opened the car door to get the items. I managed to rest all the items between my crossed arms and chest. They were placed in a tricky position.

As I walked towards the house, my worst nightmare happened. A sauce bottle slipped from my grasp and smashed all over the driveway. It startled our little girl. I could see the look on my wife's face: a look that said, *why didn't you use shopping bags?*

This situation hit me hard and quickly. I couldn't even execute this simple task. It was my first opportunity to prove myself again, and I blew it. I was one big failure and disappointment to everyone, especially myself. This was the final nail in the coffin.

All my self-hatred, failure and shame compounded at that very moment. I couldn't even talk. I jumped in my car and just drove. I didn't know where I was going. I didn't know when I was coming back. At that point, I didn't care. I was convinced the family would be better off without my negative presence around. I needed greater time to assess if this should only be my temporary viewpoint.

I spent the night a substantial distance away from home. Where I could not be located. Where no one knew where I was. I had no major possessions with me. It was a dark night, one I never want to experience again.

I did return home the next day. It was around lunch time on Friday 15 March as I waited for my wife to return from work.

* * *

That afternoon, it reached boiling point in the family kitchen. This heated conversation had been building all week. It was a delicate set of circumstances. I imagine my poor wife was trying to time this chat as best as possible. One ill-intended word, or move, could unknowingly remove the pin from the hand grenade. This hand grenade was my mind and temperament.

Things were extremely tense. My wife was now working permanently to support our family financially. She was doing all the heavy lifting. I needed to find a way to contribute to the household, marriage and our family again in a productive manner. Finding this outcome sooner rather than later was also desirable.

This is what I had to find above the surface anyway. Below the surface, the search was much deeper. I needed to decide if I wanted to choose life again, whatever life may look like moving forward.

This was a decision with serious ramifications. It could change the course of my relationships, health, wellbeing and, ultimately, life. This was not the type of decision I wanted to mess up, especially after all that had happened.

During this conversation, I vividly remember seeing the pain, suffering and tiredness all over my wife's face. I could sense she was now as broken and defeated as I was. We were both fast approaching the last station on the train line, still in a carriage together but on different seats. Plus, there was a rickety track that was shortening further by the day.

I was witnessing the anguish on someone else in a clearer light. It was not just any person; it was my greatest supporter, the one person who had always been there for me. I needed to see this and I needed to feel her pain. It was a highly charged, emotive and touching moment.

It created a spiritual experience for me. I was still stuck in the blackest of holes but, in this given moment, I was able to suddenly find a moment of instant clarity. At that exact point, I escaped my own head and decided to fight.

This fight was not for me; it was for my family. My wife and my little girl needed me. They had been there for me, and now it was my duty to do the same for them. If I was to have any hope in stepping out the other side, it had to be for them.

Following my decision to fight, a number of defining experiences shaped the next two months of my life. These events aligned like planets in the universe to set me on a path of deeper discovery. This journey would deliver lessons, wisdom and knowledge. These experiences would drive the fight further forward.

A New Game in Town

Listen to silence, it has so much to say.
– Rumi

It was a balmy summer's night. The storm had rolled in and it was now pouring down rain. My nerves were increasing – not major anxiety, like the nerves you would experience as a school student before a big exam. This was not surprising; I had literally just made my commitment to fight a few hours prior.

I scanned across the car park and could see the crowd building as I sat in the comfort of my car. There were lots of umbrellas and hurried scurrying to secure their place in line. I knew I couldn't wait any longer. I had to bite the bullet and join the crowd. I didn't want to miss out on a good seat. The people looked focused but accommodating. What did I really have to be nervous about?

My beloved Sydney City Roosters were getting ready to take on the South Sydney Rabbitohs. This was the first round of NRL in 2019. It was a game I looked forward to each year with great anticipation. Friday night football was back. What a blockbuster game it would be.

Kick off was ready and I could hear the roar of the crowd through the car radio.

STEPPING OUT THE OTHER SIDE

Shit. The Buddhist monk's address in the local community hall was also ready to start.

I quickly turned off the radio and stepped out of the car. *This better be worth it,* I thought while jogging through the rain to the front door. *I really hope none of my friends see me coming in here.*

* * *

Earlier that week, I had made a fleeting visit to our local cafe. I had picked up a flyer for an upcoming event to take place at our local community hall. A Buddhist monk was delivering a free public talk. There would be a focus on meditation. I hadn't yet made the decision to fight for life again, so I didn't pay that much attention. I mindlessly placed the flyer in the centre console when I returned to the car. It got buried among some old tax receipts and coins and I gave it no further thought.

Later that day, an old work colleague reached out over the phone. We hadn't spoken for around three years. The timing of the call was unexpected and caught me off guard. Given where my life was at, I wasn't sure what message I should communicate in a professional sense. I wasn't even sure if I was capable of having a career again. Under no circumstances would I wish to communicate that message.

I also hadn't shared my recent experience outside my very controlled inner circle. However, I did respect and trust this person. I had a sixth sense about him. Geographical and social-group distance existed between us. On this basis, it presented a safe opportunity to open up and share some minor details.

I received a pleasant response from my vulnerable sharing. Without hesitation, he told me how courageous I was. He expressed to me that I should feel proud for seeking help. I also received vulnerable insights of mental illness struggles from another perspective. The conversation was rewarding.

We discussed the benefits of meditation in detail. He had recently attended an event to listen to a Buddhist monk. The monk spoke on a range of topics, including the benefits of meditation. He confided in me that his wellbeing had improved significantly after attending this event. He also mentioned that the monk had travelled from Brisbane for the event.

The conversation politely finished. No sooner, a text message arrived with the monk's details. I had a quick read and moved on. But the universe had other ideas.

On the afternoon post deciding to fight, I went to the petrol station to fill up the car. The flyer in the car console caught my eye. *Wait a minute. It couldn't be*, I thought.

Upon further investigation, I found that it was the same Buddhist monk.

Shit. I didn't have a choice. I had to attend the event that night at the local community hall. Even if it meant missing one of the biggest games of the NRL season. Some larger force had spoken. I now needed to listen.

* * *

As I took my seat at the local community hall, I felt an element of unease. I was embarking on a new experience that was outside of my comfort zone. However, as I have come to appreciate, growth and comfort can't exist in the

39

same space. I had better become accustomed to this un-comfortable feeling if I was to move this fight forward.

The evening covered a vast number of topics and delivered valuable insights. It challenged my compromised mind, in a good way. It raised many questions around my current existential crisis. I also gained a deeper conscious awareness of how uncentred I had become.

I was lost, especially in a spiritual sense. I had no connection or reference to the wider universe. My place, among a much larger and complex system, was dislo-cated. I had been living my entire existence in my mind – a mind that had become detached from the irrefutable realities of life, a mind that had now malfunctioned one too many times.

It was both confronting and comforting that evening. Confronting in a sense that all this should have remained obvious to me. How the hell did I lose my way? Comforting in a sense that I could now relinquish the impossible battle. The universe had control, not me. My acceptance of this was well overdue.

Other than the sound of rain hitting the roof, a sooth-ing silence filled the room. My only focus was breathing. I caught a fleeting moment of tranquillity. It felt like I reconnected with a long-lost friend – a positive relation-ship that had been missing from my life and one that I longed to rekindle.

Two words stuck in my mind as I departed the local community hall that evening: curious and committed.

What other fallacies existed in my mind? Could I gain a deeper perspective around these? Would that improve my chances in the fight to step out the other side?

I was now committed to finding my centre. Mindfulness meditation would play a key role. What other tools, techniques and people could help me find my way back to myself?

I can't recall who won that game of NRL. However, the solid foundation of my newfound knowledge remains etched in my mind. For that, I am forever grateful.

Piecing a Broken Puzzle Back Together

The human brain is a complex organ with the wonderful power of enabling people to find reasons for continuing to believe whatever it is that they want to believe.

– Voltaire

It felt like we had stepped inside a high-quality design magazine. Nothing was out of place in this beautiful house. The furniture aligned at perfect angles. Everything in the kitchen was seamlessly hidden. Despite children and a resident dog, the cleanliness was immaculate.

"Wow", I overheard someone say to the owners. "The attention to detail is amazing. The interior designer has done an astonishing job. Who were they?"

"It was actually me", proclaimed one owner proudly. "It helps that I am so OCD."

That's interesting, I thought to myself. Had their mind also tricked them? Convinced them that irrational thoughts were actually real? Had they obsessed about contracting multiple life-threatening diseases? And proceeded to wash their hands compulsively to avoid such dire consequences? Or had their mind convinced them they had run someone over at night? Hit a pothole in the road while driving and then had to return to the same spot compulsively, needing to triple check no poor human was lying lifeless on the bitumen?

Luckily, common sense would prevail. I kept my thoughts to myself, before making a total dick of myself or making others feel extremely uncomfortable. Welcome to the complex world of obsessive-compulsive disorder – a world that shares very little with 'being so OCD', for clarification.

In modern times, the reference made to being 'so OCD' is common. It has become part of the vernacular. It can explain a range of personality traits, such as a desire for cleanliness or order. Some of these behaviours are no doubt productive in certain instances.

Previously, I wouldn't have given this specific use of terminology a second thought. This has changed some-what post medical diagnosis for my obsessive-compulsive disorder. It is something I have become more attuned to recognising.

I am not on a personal crusade to educate people on their own choice of words. It is merely an interest-ing observable pattern of modern human behaviour. This observation of wider society has forced me to examine my own internal dialogue, particularly my beliefs, percep-tions and choice of words around mental illness.

* * *

Post deciding to fight, I made some significant commit-ments. One of these was to take greater responsibility around my mental illness. This was a non-negotiable be-tween me and my family.

An accurate diagnosis was now in place. This provided a much-needed level of certainty to take two critical steps forward. These steps were big rocks. They were foundational steps for putting the broken puzzle back together.

Step one: take personal responsibility for my learning. I wanted to know everything possible about obsessive-compulsive disorder.

Step two: place the right support network around me, a network that would exist on a consistent and ongoing basis.

It was a monumental decision to accept that I needed others to proactively assist with the fight. The time spent in hospital, broken, had convinced me. I had proven that I wasn't capable of navigating these rough waters by myself. Bandaid fixes and a reactive approach was no longer a viable option.

Step one would be less challenging. I was in full control of this outcome. Step two was not as straightforward. We needed to identify a psychologist who specialised in obsessive-compulsive disorder and had availability to take on a new patient.

The best medical specialists always have long waiting lists. It was a benefit that I no longer had time pressure in a traditional sense. But each day spent in my current state without professional support was a risk.

* * *

I was surprised to discover that a clinic specialising in obsessive-compulsive disorder was close by. It was actually located in the same suburb as our family home. I would have driven past this building twice a day for a period of seven years. I had never paid enough attention to notice. The somewhat ironic lesson in this is now not lost on me. No longer will I view my mental illness as being out of sight, then also out of mind.

My psychiatrist referred me to this clinic. The head doctor was a revered psychologist, one who specialised in obsessive-compulsive disorder. As expected, a doctor of this calibre was not in a position to be taking on new patients.

Thankfully, the doctor decided to make time available for me in her lunch hour every Friday. I guess my recent hospitalisation influenced the decision or, perhaps, the delicate situation around my wellbeing. Either way, to find myself in this fortunate position was a blessing.

I am not a trained medical professional. Therefore, I won't go into the specifics used in these clinical sessions. It would be irresponsible on my behalf. However, it is important to disclose one detail. Outside of my wife, the psychologist was my next critical support person. They both kept me on track through this challenging period. The psychologist's role was tricky: she had to try to keep everything balanced, often on a very slippery slope.

This experience provided much greater value to me than I had anticipated. For me, it was more than a psychologist treating a mental illness in a clinical manner. It helped build my knowledge around the scientific aspects of my brain. It provided a professional perspective that I respected. It gave me comfort that my battle was real and challenging. What I had been trying to conquer and achieve was a sizeable mountain peak.

Most importantly, it helped me restore some self-love and appreciation. I needed this more than anything at this stage of my journey. The psychologist believed in me, when I still didn't. She made a commitment to work with me on an ongoing basis. No matter how busy she was, she always made time during her lunch break. She was also not afraid to respectfully challenge me – always from a position of care and only when I needed it.

* * *

Sometimes, I am asked to explain obsessive-compulsive disorder. I always deliver a response that is not overtly clinical or complicated. The concept of a brain lock is what appears to resonate well with most people. The concept is covered in greater detail in a book called *Brain Lock* – a book written by an American psychiatrist called Jeffrey Schwartz.

For example, if I was planning to leave my house to go to work, the front part of my brain would logically communicate that I need to close and lock the front door. If I was in a healthy functioning state, I would move the message from the front region of my brain to the central region of my brain. It would communicate that the door was locked. I could then move forward with my next task on the way to work.

My brain, suffering from obsessive-compulsive disorder, could respond differently. Despite locking the door successfully, it would not transfer the message as required. The front region of the brain fails to communicate with the central region of the brain. The message becomes locked and on repeat loop, like an obsession. As a result, I will continue to compulsively keep checking and relocking the door.

I know the door has been locked. This is rational. Unfortunately, my faulty brain wiring results in the irrational behaviour of rechecking. A key factor in this faulty wiring is a lack of serotonin in my brain. This chemical enables the communication of brain messages as required. Simplistically, a chemical imbalance exists in my brain.

* * *

I have learned significant detail about obsessive-compulsive disorder. I now understand how my brain functions differently. One vital learning point about the disorder and my brain stands out above everything else. Academic research published in the July 2016 edition of the scientific journal *Molecular Psychiatry* found that obsessive-compulsive disorder sufferers are ten times more likely to commit suicide than the general population.

Recent scientific studies of obsessive-compulsive disorder have advanced. There is greater detail around the real challenges sufferers can face. This presents a level of risk that makes me sit up and pay close attention. It ensures I now have no choice in managing my mental illness. A proactive plan that consists of ongoing, regular visits to my psychologist is a must. Transparent, honest engagement with my wider support network is also a must. Such decisions and choices could have unintended life or death repercussions.

This knowledge has also helped me to better contextualise my sudden hospitalisation. The hospitalisation was a gift in the context of any potential alternative. I still shoulder some guilt around this situation and who I let down – in particular, my family. It is not uncommon to wake up some mornings with sickness in the pit of my stomach. Sickness that comes from past shame. However, this has decreased over time, given my understanding of what was really at stake.

It is often said that knowledge is power. I now had a far better understanding of the science around my mental illness. I also had the right professional support network in place. These were significant steps forward. However, an intense level of self-work was still required in the fight.

Finding the most intricate piece of the puzzle required deeper searching. Fighting for our family had initially gotten me back off the canvas. Now the fight needed to move through the middle rounds. To do this, I needed to fight for myself again. This was imperative for my healing process and self-evolution.

Even Red Roses Cast Dark Shadows – The Shadow Part 1

Seek the wisdom that will untie your knot. Seek the path that demands your whole being.
– Rumi

I was not built for boxing; my height-to-weight ratio couldn't be any less favourable. But I love the sport. Nothing signifies greater physical and mental strength than boxing. Prior to my hospitalisation, it is now evident that my shadow was regularly writing cheques that my body simply could never cash.

On one particularly fateful day, I was struggling to stand up. Every limb was aching. My breath was gone. I had even dry retched in the corner of the boxing gym. What I needed was water and a rest. Finding someone prepared to tell me the truth was never an easy task.

The hour-long session was nearing its end. My friend, a fit man and more than capable boxer, approached from a position of care. He could see I was most likely a danger to myself if I continued any further. He politely informed me that I should take it easy on the last exercise.

He insinuated I shouldn't jump over the small obstacles that were set out in a straight line; it would be wiser if I ran around them instead. This set a fire off inside; it was like a red rag to a bull. I less-than-politely insinuated back that he could piss off. I would be jumping over those obstacles if it was the last thing I did. I only made it to the third obstacle. I clipped it and fell. I landed on my ankle and broke it. I hobbled out of the gym, unaided of course.

I felt like I may have lost the battle, but I had been victorious in the war. Anyone else in the gym, including my friend, probably wished I would slow the hell down. There was no battle or war to win that day, apart from the dangerous ones that had manifested in my head again.

My ankle took a long time to heal, much longer than it should have. Despite medical advice and my wife's frustrations, I refused to use crutches. Another battle, and war, fought and won. At least, I thought so anyway.

The real enemy was far more covert. It were invisible, dangerous and entrenched deep in my subconscious. It was laughing as it slaughtered me consistently across all key battle fronts. I never had an answer, and this sneaky enemy wanted to keep it that way.

In hindsight, this day at the gym is just one example of many where my shadow was at work.

* * *

After the Buddhist monk evening, I had made the commitment to reconnect with my centre. I started to examine a variety of tools and techniques I might use for benefit.

I was aware of a duality that exists everywhere in life, especially given the yin-yang concept rooted in the philosophy of Taoism. Where good exists, bad is also present. Black cannot exist without white. Death always concludes life's journey.

However, I had limited exposure to the shadow side through the duality concept. I had some exposure through brand architypes, characters found in stories and song lyrics. In terms of the power of the shadow, from a psychological growth perspective, I knew little. This was all about to change. To recentre myself as desired, I would require a deeper understanding of my own shadow side.

I knew this would not be a pleasant experience and not just because of the raw emotions of my current state of mind and recent events. There is a good reason why the shadow is rarely covered in self-development material. People are never going to find it enjoyable to deeply examine their shortcomings, especially when the alternative is to assess their strengths and bask in their glory. People go to great lengths to protect their self-image, especially from anything unfamiliar or uncomfortable that challenges their own personal story – a story that enables the masking of their shadow.

I was under no illusions; this was going to be hard work. But I had chosen to fight for myself and for the girls. The hardest fight one can have is the one against themselves. I needed to have this internal fight.

I had also discovered that the shadow can be a complex psychological concept, typically communicated in a manner that is not easily digestible. I eventually enrolled in an online course delivered by an organisation named CEOsage. This course was called 'Shadow Training, Getting to Know and Integrate Your Shadow'.

* * *

The course was exceptional. It delivered high-quality content that was applicable in the modern world. It was accessible and practical. It was so beneficial that I made a request to share some of the content from the course in this book. This request was kindly granted.

In a basic sense, the shadow is a psychological term for everything that people can't see in themselves. It represents the dark side of a person's personality. It consists of primitive, negative emotions and impulses. It represents the parts of people they no longer claim to be their own. These unexamined or disowned parts of the personality never leave. Instead, they find a way to hide.

Everyone carries a shadow. It is not the shadow's existence that generates challenges. It is when the shadow is ignored and not integrated that real problems can manifest.

Every young child has basic human needs. These include physiological safety, security, and a need for belonging. As children grow, traits associated with being good are accepted. These traits are positively reinforced. Other traits, often associated with being bad, are rejected.

Children grow to express certain parts of themselves. Depending on their expression, they can receive negative cues from their environment. Often this process may threaten one of their basic needs. For instance, constant disapproval from parents or teachers can threaten a child's security. Likewise, ridicule from classmates can threaten a child's sense of belonging.

Children learn to adjust their behaviour to match their needs. They learn to adapt to their external world. Through this process of adaption, all the rejected and discouraged components become hidden. This takes place during a child's formative, middle and adolescent years. The rejected parts form a shadow.

Despite this process, the shadow remains ingrained in the subconscious. In the absence of any conscious awareness, this shadow can wreak havoc. Patterns of self-sabotaging behaviour or blind spots can emerge. People often remain oblivious to these unproductive behaviours.

As a result, people are more attuned at identifying and observing the shadow of others. People identify in others the exact qualities they try so hard to deny and hide in themselves. Projection is the psychological term given to this behaviour.

In a close relationship, one partner may subconsciously hide their anger. This anger becomes further suppressed as life evolves. Heated arguments regularly take place in the relationship. Both partners contribute equally to these arguments. The partner with the suppressed anger and shadow may view the other as an antagonistic tyrant. Ironically, they may see themselves as the calmer, innocent participant.

Upon conclusion of the Shadow Work course, plus the intense process of examining every piece of myself (the good, bad and indifferent), I developed a conscious awareness of the following points:

- I had been denying my shadow for 38 years of my life.

- I had been hiding my shadow at every opportunity I could.
- I had been lying to myself and others to keep my shadow from appearing.
- I had a belief system and internal story that shamed my shadow.
- I had been projecting my shadow onto others.
- I had not lived life to its full potential because of my shadow.
- I had almost paid the ultimate price due, in part, to my shadow.

My shadow is not my mental illness, now diagnosed as obsessive-compulsive disorder.

My shadow was my own cruel perception of my mental illness until diagnosis.

I had been running away from my shadow for far too long, looking to put in place bandaid fixes at every opportunity. Everything was directed toward never having to own, or disclose, my mental illness.

The full integration of my shadow into life was now business critical. Otherwise, I would never find my centre. Only a whole person could move the fight forward. The true version of myself needed to stand up. Taking full responsibility for my shadow integration process was solely on my shoulders. This was within my circle of control, which provided comfort.

During the Shadow Work course, I read that the great philosopher Alan Watts once mentioned, nothing exists on the dark side of which to be afraid; once this is accepted, all that remains is love.

I wanted to feel this love again. Not love from others – I was grateful to already be surrounded by this in spades. I needed to find love for myself again. I had fought one too many unnecessary battles and wars in my mind. I was well overdue to put down the imaginary weapons.

Icarus and the Sun
– The Shadow Part 2

Never regret thy fall, O Icarus of the fearless flight.
For the greatest tragedy of them all, is never to feel the
burning light.
– Oscar Wilde

I can remember our family's white Mitsubishi Magna passing various bus shelters. They overflowed with excited children waiting to go to school. They all looked happy enough. Some were even playing games. This all baffled me, especially given I was on a mission – a mission to stay away from school at all costs that day.

Mum was driving. My brother was in the front and I was in the back, wishing I could just disappear from the whole situation. The tension was high. My downright refusal to attend school had taken its toll on the family already that day. I had to be physically forced into the car with tears flowing.

We now had to drive my brother to high school. He had missed his bus thanks to my less than desirable carry on. He was no doubt adjusting to a foreign and challenging period in his own life. The last thing he would have needed was his little brother making things more difficult.

Everyone was quiet; a knife could have cut the air. The radio was on louder than usual, most likely to drown out any profanities I would callously direct towards the front of the car at will.

Boom, crack. Boom, crack! Crash! This sound blared from the radio. It filled the void of silence that lingered throughout the car. It was the opening drum fill for the Phil Collins song, *I Wish It Would Rain Down.*

Still to this very day, I develop an almost instant feeling of sadness whenever I hear this song. My eyes start to well up. Deep in my chest and stomach, I get a strange sensation. It is a reminder of how I felt during the first breakdown in my life.

Maybe it's a reminder of what others experienced when supporting me through a breakdown, what my family would have experienced during this challenging time. It's also a reminder of how wonderful my family are, how much my family cares, and how my family did everything to help me with my mental illness. They left no stone unturned.

* * *

I had an exceptional upbringing in a loving family household. I could not have wished for anything more. However, like everyone, I still have a shadow. And, upon deeper reflection, it was most likely created in my middle childhood years, around the time when *I Wish It Would Rain Down* was being played on the radio.

My mental illness first showed signs of existence between the ages of eight and eleven. I missed an extended period of school in year five. This resulted from a series of unproductive obsessive thoughts, obsessive thoughts that I could not control. Irrational and scary thoughts that my young mind mistook as reality.

On multiple occasions, I convinced myself I was suffering from a life-threatening disease. Most children at this young age would not have even heard of such diseases. As soon as I felt I had avoided one disease, I would move on to stressing about the next. To try and avoid these fabricated diseases, I would wash my hands compulsively. Consequently, during this period of life, my fingers resembled the outer texture of a prune more often than not.

My caring, loving and supportive parents took me to a range of medical professionals. They drove all over town to seek help. Their hard work paid dividends. I got through this initial challenging period at a young age. I managed to continue through the best part of the next decade without another major breakdown. From a medical perspective, all appeared to have worked perfectly.

Detailed shadow work has shed greater perspective on this critical period. It influenced my own personal psychological development. This could not be avoided. About thirty years have now passed. But I can still recall the various psychologists centres we attended. The locations and faces of the doctors are still etched in my memory.

I was well aware that my parents were having to take time out of their work to attend these appointments with me. I also knew my older brother, three years my senior, never burdened my parents with any of these types of issues. None of my young friends were having to attend such intense medical appointments, not to my knowledge anyway, nor were they downright refusing to go to school. They all seemed balanced, not shit scared of imaginative events that had no connection to reality.

I often envied other children during this critical period of time in my life. I wished I could be more like them. I perceived them to be carefree. My perception was that they didn't have to deal with psychological challenges like I did.

What I was experiencing growing up was not exactly the same as others, at least in my own mind. My sense of belonging, as it related to my peer group, was different. The impact of these events was magnified, purely because of the important age bracket in which they occurred.

Guilt, shame, embarrassment and inferiority ran riot during this period. A short, three-year timeframe would have longer lasting implications in life. My ego had now been firmly fixed. It was put in place to protect me from anything that would ever make me feel different or inferior to my peers in the future.

The conscious brain played its role perfectly. It pushed these painful events and feelings deep into the subconscious. This created a shadow. The shadow would keep the pain associated with these feelings well hidden, away from everyone and everything, for as long as possible. From this moment forward, the subconscious rarely missed a beat. It helped me to develop textbook patterns of behaviour to protect my self-image. It kept the shadow hidden deeply within.

The subconscious crafted a devious plan. It consistently reinforced to me and others that the shadow didn't exist. I consciously played a key role. I would look for any opportunity to prove that I was mentally strong. I could match it with the 'tough ones', so to speak. I would push myself to the highest levels possible. This way I could keep it hidden from everyone that I battled with mental illness. My internal perception was that high performing individuals were always mentally strong. They rarely displayed weakness. I needed to be one of them; no one would ever suspect a thing if I operated at their level.

Pushing myself to perform at this level was downright irresponsible, especially in the context of my mental illness. I was the only person responsible for this. I would like to say that the hindsight bias exists on this front, but it doesn't. I needed to crash, burn and fall spectacularly hard from grace. I could not develop a conscious awareness of this pattern through any other means. This helps contextualise the power of the shadow if left unattended.

People who cared for my wellbeing often tried to show me another way, tried to help me see I needed to slow down or balance out my life. Embarrassingly, these people were often met with my disdain. It would light a fire deep inside. I would double down and emerge like a competitive beast. I needed to prove them wrong, to throw them off the scent of my shadow. In this regard, there were periods of my life where I would distance myself from others, especially if I thought they were starting to get too close. They were a risk that needed managing if they had seen glimpses of my shadow.

I compare the famous story of Icarus, Daedalus and the sun to my patterns – my self-sabotaging, unproductive and dangerous patterns of behaviour. Daedalus, the father of Icarus, told his son to fly within the extremes of the sun and the water. Icarus ignored the wisdom of Daedalus, soaring high towards the sun. The heat from the sun melted the wax on the wings and Icarus plunged into the ocean.

Unlike Icarus, I had touched the outskirts of the sun previously. My wings were singed or broken, but they were repairable. This enabled flight to take place again. The dangerous, self-sabotage patterns of behaviour could repeat themselves.

The internal story ingrained in my subconscious was powerful. It needed to keep shooting for the sun; otherwise, I was mentally weak and not good enough to belong within my peer group. I subconsciously wanted to be like the highest of achievers. And they were always seeking the extremities of the sun. During my existential crisis, I didn't just touch the outskirts of the sun; I went headfirst into the centre. And, just like Icarus, I was badly burnt and fell.

The key lesson from Icarus, Daedalus and the sun is straightforward: stick to the middle and avoid the extremes, otherwise known as remaining balanced. Sadly, Icarus never got another chance. I still had one. I needed to fight hard not to mess it up.

The brutal reality was not lost on me. This may be my final chance if I didn't find a way to put proactive mechanisms in place to sustain balance in my life. I needed to prove I was capable of this to those I had hurt most when I had fallen. They needed to see I was capable of remaining balanced in the future. I needed a life with greater balance. More importantly, so did the girls. This meant the role I played in our life moving forward needed to evolve. This was non-negotiable from a family perspective – the only perspective that now mattered.

Old Dog Learns New Tricks

Well-being is attained little by little, and nevertheless
is no little thing itself.
– Zeno of Citium

One of my fondest childhood memories is of visiting the museum. The boys in our family were all dinosaur mad. It provided the perfect place for us to burn off energy on holidays. We would spend hours examining fossils, climbing all over life-sized replica models and fighting over who earned the right to be T-Rex on the way home.

I had always longed for the day when I could return to the museum and relive some of those positive memories and good times. I woke up one Thursday in late April 2019 and decided to make this happen.

Thursdays had become the day I shared alone with our little girl. They were now vastly different to the Thursdays before my hospitalisation. This was traditionally the day where I would examine every newspaper possible, often like a person possessed, transferring all financial and property information from print into my mind. This activity no longer formed any part of my new Thursday regime.

I would love to be able to say I was a natural at parenting, but I wasn't. It took me some time to adjust to full days with my little one. So, when I decided we would visit the museum together, I thought I may have bitten off more than I could chew.

I first had to share the idea with my wife. Trust is a disproportionate beast. It takes a long time to build but is lost in the blink of an eye. Rebuilding trust with the girls had now become a core focus in my fight. I was, therefore, very relieved when my wife was supportive of my idea.

This was a special moment for me. It was the first sign that I was moving in the right direction for our family. In many ways, it was the ultimate sign of my wife's trust: allowing me to take our most precious gift out into the real world alone.

* * *

It turned out that our sweet, little three-year-old girl didn't share my same love of dinosaurs. Truth be told, she was shit scared. This was not the only parenting lesson I learned during that day.

A cafe caught the eye of my little girl. It was getting close to lunch time, so it made sense to stop. It also provided another father and daughter bonding opportunity. I may have needed to make up some lost ground post the whole dinosaur fiasco.

While ordering our lunch at the counter, I noticed my little girl wandering calmly to a close-by table to sit down. I remember thinking that it was very confident behaviour for a three-year-old. I waited for our lunch and kept a close eye on the table. Every time our eyes met, I was rewarded with a gorgeous little cheeky smile. The lady serving me commented on how beautiful she was and that butter wouldn't melt in her mouth. I nodded in agreement.

I finally made it to the table with our lunch. I reached out to place an apple juice in my girl's left hand. As I did this, she sheepishly transferred something from her left hand to her right. "What was that?" I asked. She just returned another one of those butter-wouldn't-melt-in-your-mouth smiles.

Upon further investigation, I found a half-eaten packet of Mentos lollies. Talk about a fast moving and opportunistic child. The old me would have become frustrated, hurriedly disciplined my little one, paid for the lollies and apologised profusely. But this provided me with an opportunity, a chance to demonstrate that I could parent in a calmer and, hopefully, more productive manner.

I now had extra bandwidth. My mind was not over-loaded with such irrational, obsessive and unproductive thoughts. I could take my time to talk to my little one and try to meet her at her level. I could communicate in a calmer, more balanced manner, explaining why this behaviour was not acceptable. We even went and apologised to the lady behind the counter together. Needless to say, the lady and I both now understood the cheeky smiles we'd received.

Overall, the day at the museum was a beautiful experience. It provided a glimpse into my future: a more balanced future. It was a future I was capable of embracing, a future I was starting to believe I was worthy of experiencing.

* * *

Self-work focused on recentring and the shadow made me question such worthiness. It was glaringly obvious that I had not been consistent in my congruency. My behaviour had not always been in line with what I perceived to be my core values.

For instance, on Thursday mornings in the past, my family's expectations around me pulling my weight as a parent had slowly deteriorated. In fact, they would generally just stay out of my way. I was only interested in one thing, obsessively reading newspapers. I was probably best described as 'persona non grata' when I became immersed in such obsessive states.

My conscious brain could quickly and confidently articulate my values. Family was always my number one value and priority. However, the subconscious would override any rational thought process. It would take control and ensure any decisions made would be in the best interests of hiding my shadow.

This would manifest in real life as a distinctive pattern. I would often make decisions that put my career, or my own need to achieve, ahead of my family. Often, these were not logical decisions driven by any form of rational thought. There was no external pressure applied. It was all self-inflicted. The ego would protect the shadow and its associated insecurities.

This non-congruence between my behaviour and values was frustrating for loved ones. It would have been difficult to watch and comprehend. I am ashamed to admit that sometimes, after work, I would book a hotel room. I wouldn't tell anyone. I would do this so I could continue to work longer, as opposed to attending to my responsibilities on the family front. I would never end up staying the night. At around 11 pm, the conscious brain would resume some form of control and I would return to the family home.

Significant work on my part was required to demonstrate to my girls that I could improve on this front. To evolve into a family role that would better align my behaviour with my values. This was not an easy process. I likened it to an old dog having to learn new tricks. This is not impossible, but it was never going to be straightforward. It would take concerted time, effort and growth.

* * *

I had never been one to get excited about grocery shopping. I was even less enthralled about having to create lists and prepare for the process. Like multiple parts of my life, it was undertaken like a race. Get in, get it done as fast as possible, and get out. Then get on to something else that I perceived as being more important or productive.

I was now responsible for the family's entire food and grocery requirements every week. Learning a better, more effective way to shop was imperative. Further to this, my exposure to major public places with people had been limited. Grocery shopping would be a substantial challenge and sizeable achievement for me. This puts some perspective on how broken I was. It also provided an opportunity to demonstrate that I was attempting to make progress in creating newfound balance between my behaviour and my values.

I toyed with the idea that I should just order the groceries online. This would avoid any likely triggers of anxiety or negative self-belief. However, this would have been short-sighted behaviour. Such decision-making would not demonstrate to myself or the girls that I had the fight in me, the fight to deliver on my agreed responsibilities for our family.

I also revisited my existing frame of the entire grocery shopping journey. Given I was no longer time poor, grocery shopping provided a perfect environment, an environment where I could put into action some of my recent techniques and learnings – concepts I had acquired from time in hospital, psychologist appointments, and my own self-discovery.

Grocery shopping needed to evolve. In the past, pure mindlessness describes my routine accurately. It evolved to a mindful experience grounded in the present moment. I would walk down every aisle, even those in which I didn't need to purchase anything. All I focused on was my breathing, posture and executing the task at hand.

When I arrived at the check-out, bandwidth even remained for me to engage in meaningful conversations. I would converse with people behind the registers about their day and life in general. One lady even used to compliment me, amazed that I undertook the shopping for our family every week. She insinuated with a wry smile that her husband was not capable. At times, I came close to explaining to her why I had taken up such responsibility.

Grocery shopping also enabled the creation of a beautiful little bonding ritual for our family. After each shop, I would depart with a handful of little toys – a complimentary bonus: toys from the movie *The Lion King*. Whenever I picked up our little girl from day care, I also had a new *Lion King* toy in my pocket. The surprise was always met with a look of pure joy and delight from my little one.

The simple act of grocery shopping signified so much to me and my family. It became a weekly ritual that I learned to embrace and look forward to. It was a small step forward in feeling productive and purposeful again. It felt like an eternity waiting for this uplifting experience. Most importantly, it enabled me to start to reconnect with my beautiful family again. The reality was that this small step forward had created an overall larger ripple effect. It had given me the confidence to branch out further and seek even greater purpose.

* * *

Meals on Wheels was a charity I supported when I was a teenager. When I made a decision to start giving back to the community, it was the first organisation that came to mind. I commenced assisting the local Meals on Wheels almost immediately, a couple of times a week. This moment was a game changer. It was clear evidence that my mental health and wellbeing was improving. It was also a sign that I was beginning to live my values again, by putting the needs of others with challenges ahead of my own.

From my experience, mental illnesses require a very inward-focused battle. External perspective sadly disappears, as the pure instinct for self-survival takes over. I find this one of the hardest things to rationalise in my own mind about my mental illness. When healthy, I place a high personal value on assisting others. While I can't be all things to all people, I do try my best to improve my empathy skills. I may never find total comfort around my own perceived selfishness with mental illness. Guilt and shame always rise to the surface when I simply can't be there for others when needing to save myself. However, as I am constantly reminded by my support team, I am no good to anyone if I don't prioritise care of myself when it is required.

Shifting my focus outwardly at this point was a defining moment in the fight. I was ready to give back to the community and people in need, people in much greater need than myself, as my health and wellbeing improved.

I was slowly taking small steps toward becoming a productive member of our family and the community once again. However, I was still living a somewhat sheltered existence. I was free from major triggers and temptations to encourage my destructive behavioural patterns. This was all about to change. Change was being forced upon me, given I needed to find a way to contribute financially to our family again.

I was just starting to adjust to my version of a new reality, but this wasn't a viable long-term solution. I needed to step back out into the real world again. I needed to find an even greater level of courage and tenacity. The fight was being taken deeper. I was headed into the championship rounds.

SECTION THREE

Stepping Out

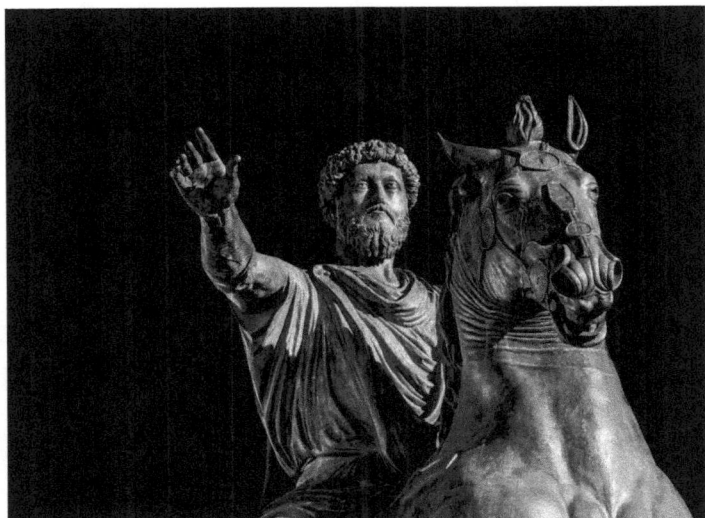

At dawn, when you have trouble getting out of bed
Tell yourself: I have to go to work—as a human being
What do I have to complain of,
if I'm going to do what I was born for?
The things I was brought into the world to do?
Or is this what I was created for?
To huddle under the blankets and stay warm?
Don't you see the plants, the birds,
the ants and spiders and bees
Going about their individual tasks, putting the world
in order, as best they can?
And you're not willing to do your job
as a human being?
Why aren't you running to do what
your nature demands?
– Marcus Aurelius

I remember turning to my friend and stating in pure disbelief, "He's dead". No human could survive that onslaught. I have never seen the back of a person's head hit the canvas so hard. It must have landed with a thud. It may leave a divot in the ring, like a shotput does after it lands on an athletics track. Tyson Fury couldn't die now. He was just on the comeback trail. He had a young family. We felt we were watching a live tragedy in the making.

Tyson Fury had taken two flush punches on the chin. One sent him falling towards the canvas. The second, shockingly, caught him on the way down. He was most likely knocked out already when the final punch landed.

These were not standard punches. They were from a man who knocked out almost everyone who dared enter the ring with him. His punching power was second to none. Deontay Wilder was deadly, and he had just fired his most potent weapons. No human could survive this. But Tyson Fury is not your average human. Consequently, he got back up.

It was not an average human who rose from the canvas that night. It was not an average human who made the referees count. It was not an average human who finished the fight stronger than his opponent.

Tyson Fury had fought back from depression; he was suicidal at his lowest point. When he rose from the canvas that night, he made it clear that his miracle performance was to inspire others battling with mental health challenges. He encouraged people like myself not to give up.

It is said that inspiration can be found in the most unlikely of places.

A charismatic heavyweight boxer and a philosophy founded in the early 3rd century BC may not seem to have much in common. Boxers are not traditionally associated with delivering life-altering wisdom, while philosophers excel in this space. Differences aside, Tyson Fury and Stoicism were both sources of inspiration, enabling me to take my fight through the deeper rounds.

The world heavyweight boxing champion is often regarded as the strongest and most dangerous man on the planet. One of the greatest heavyweight champions of this generation also battles mental illness. He has become an unlikely ambassador, following his own personal battles.

Tyson Fury's fall from grace and subsequent comeback is extremely well documented. His journey will remain one of the greatest stories in sporting history. The timing of his unfortunate battle and recovery was fortuitous for me. It provided me with the exact inspiration I needed. It gave me strength and provided encouragement that I would be able to integrate back into society at a fully functioning level.

Tyson Fury has commented that beating his mental illness was the toughest battle he has had to endure.

When the best heavyweight boxer in the world said this, I listened. I was blown away. It helped move the needle for my own confidence, courage and commitment. It inspired me to keep fighting and reframe my perceived weakness as strength.

It is the duality of Tyson Fury that I find so appealing. He does punch people for a living. But he also displays a softer and empathetic caring side. He is proud and vulnerable to show this side of himself. He owns all of himself; he doesn't run away from his shadow. He has made mistakes, said things he possibly wishes he hadn't. Tyson Fury is like every other human; he is real.

It is fair to say, for an extended period of time, I lived, ate and breathed all things Tyson Fury. I would watch videos of Tyson Fury training, his ring walks, his interviews. I even listened to the same songs he liked. I studied this man closely from a distance. His vulnerable and brutally honest story, warts and all, gave me hope and self-belief.

* * *

Alongside Tyson Fury, Stoicism also delivered hope for a better future. Cognitive Behavioural Therapy was a technique I was taught by my support team of medical professionals. It assists in managing my obsessive-compulsive disorder. I actively searched for further readings on Cognitive Behavioural Therapy; I wanted to learn more. I was deeply intrigued when references were regularly made to the ancient philosophy of Stoicism. I had a basic understanding of the philosophy and its principles. It had become modernised to an extent through a series of popular and user-friendly books – books I had now read.

What I did not fully appreciate, however, were the deep links to psychology. A strong focus on controlling non-productive thoughts exists in Stoicism. It encourages a healthier and more tranquil mindset. Stoicism provided the perfect antidote I needed. It helped stop me from slipping back into historical faulty thinking patterns. I had the ability to call upon a time-tested philosophy, one that deeply aligned with how I needed to evolve. This was invaluable given real-world triggers were about to consistently fly at me again.

Philosophy is often misunderstood as a purely intellectual pursuit. I, for one, had certainly been guilty of this wrongful assessment in the past. I have learned this is not the case with Stoicism. I can apply the principles and learnings in the real world for genuine benefit. This is something I have now come to deeply value about Stoicism. I don't need a deep theoretical understanding of this philosophy. I can take what I learn and generate positive impacts in my life.

Stoicism helped me gain greater conscious awareness, especially around a number of fallacies that existed in my mind. I had wrongfully accepted most of these as gospel. I was never courageous enough to challenge such beliefs.

I may never be able to voluntarily control my mental illness, particularly not without the assistance of medication and my close support network. However, I can take greater personal responsibility for matters where I control the circumstances. The proactive practice of Stoicism has made a material difference to my life in this regard.

It is now apparent that I had lost faith in the universe. I could not see a better future. I had given up on myself. Stoicism helped rekindled my faith. I would not have been prepared to step back into the real world, as quickly as I did, without it. Further to this, I certainly would not have had the courage and self-belief to pivot my career, especially in the context of my extreme loss of confidence, identity and self-worth.

There were five key insights that enabled me to move through the deeper rounds of the fight. They enabled me to stay standing on my own two feet until the penultimate round. These insights – listed below – were often shaped by the principles and learnings of Stoicism.

Insight 1 – Apply a Broader Lens – Empathy

Insight 2 – Own All of It – Shadow Integration

Insight 3 – Not Everything Ages Like Fine Wine – Beliefs

Insight 4 – The Fallacy of Control – Create My Certainty

Insight 5 – What You Do Have – Gratitude

Apply a Broader Lens – Empathy

Could a greater miracle take place than for us to look through each other's eyes for an instant?
– Henry David Thoreau

In May 2019, I returned back to paid work. I started again at my previous place of employment. I was going back in a much less strenuous capacity for obvious reasons. Hindsight is a wonderful thing. With an accurate diagnosis in place, it was evident that my previous role was not the right fit for me.

I liken the previous role to competing in a series of sprint races, every day, with a faulty hamstring. Some days, the hamstring would hold up fine. I could finish all the races. Other times, my hamstring would remain ruptured for days, or weeks. I would have to fight like anything just to keep it in an operational state, let alone work out how to finish the races. It was a consistent, added burden to carry through all the sprint races. This eventually took its toll.

Armed with new information, I am surprised I managed to perform my previous role for the length of time I did. These so-called sprint races are often silent battles. They are rarely fully understood or appreciated.

In my opinion, mental illness and mental health are two separate concepts. Everybody has to make wise and conscious choices to manage their own mental health. There is an element of self-control and personal responsibility in influencing one's own mental health. In contrast, exceptional mental health management won't always avert a mental illness. The illness can develop beyond a person's control, desire and avoidance effort.

For instance, I could practice the best mental health care routine. This may include eating a cleaner diet, balanced exercise, no alcohol and optimistic thinking, just to name a few obvious examples. In my experience, however, exemplary mental health management will not always avert my mental illness challenges, especially if I look to fight against, or avoid, other routines that can be perceived as less than favourable for a variety of reasons.

Taking regular medication is one such routine. No one ever wants to take medication if they don't need to; I personally fought against this for a very long time. But in my specific set of circumstances, medication must form one critical part of a multifaceted approach to managing my mental illness. It took a long time to shift my beliefs on this front. However, I now perceive that any potential side effects resulting from taking medication are a small price to pay if the outcome is that I remain on this earth in a functioning state for our family.

* * *

Deep down, I was shit scared about returning to work. What would people think of me? How would I avoid the triggers and not make the same painful mistakes again?

Could I even perform a role that added value to the organisation any longer?

The organisation was kind and enabled me to return two days a week to a lesser role. This was a gesture for which our family will always remain extremely grateful. This return meant so much more than just an opportunity to contribute again to our family financially. It was a critical component of my healing process.

I had been a leader for an extended period of time at this organisation. This was a role that I'd shouldered with the responsibility and respect it deserved. As a leader, I always encouraged two key principles in people I had the pleasure of leading. One was to show empathy to others. The other was not to be afraid to show personal vulnerability.

It was not lost on me that real leadership is not about a position or title. It is a deliberate choice in behaviour and attitude. Anyone can be a leader. Leaders are also human; they can fall from grace and shouldn't be afraid to share their honest learnings if this occurs.

I was certainly no longer a leader by title or position. But I still had a responsibility as a leader to show up and set an example. I had to find the courage to see past my own feelings of shame and embarrassment. A broader lens was required for the situation. I would only get through this if I made this about others by focusing on something far greater than myself.

My experience would have impacted other people in different ways. I needed to show empathy and vulnerability towards others. This was the right thing to do. I had to reframe the set of events as an opportunity to grow. Growth and comfort can never exist in the same space. I knew I couldn't avoid feeling uncomfortable in this situation, especially if I was going to approach it like a real leader should and put my ego to the side.

The organisation had kindly offered the opportunity for me to undertake my new role from home. However, my medical support team was confident that I was ready to face reality again. They believed I could negate any triggers that may arise. I would need to put appropriate boundaries in place to remain balanced, boundaries that I placed on myself for the most part. There was no reason why I couldn't attempt to face this head on.

Re-engaging with work colleagues face-to-face was important to me. These were great people. I didn't want anyone to feel like they should have seen the warning signs before my fall. No one had forward visibility on the complex reality of my situation, not even me or my family. This all changed once I spent valuable time in hospital. An accurate diagnosis would confirm that my fast and unpredictable fall was a result of my mental illness.

I needed to empathise with what this may have felt like on the other side of the fence. It would have been a confronting process. I made the decision to be vulnerable. I would disclose, to anyone who was interested, the full diagnosis of my mental illness. This would include my ongoing management plan. I needed to be upfront that I was taking appropriate medication and seeking ongoing medical support. In light of my transparency and vulnerability, people were very caring and supportive upon my return.

* * *

Diabetes Australia reports that 1.7 million Australians (6.7%) have diabetes. In contrast, the Australian National Survey of Mental Health and Wellbeing reports that 20% of Australians (5.1 million) will have, or develop, a mental illness. Countless more will struggle to maintain their general mental health. This quantifies the magnitude of the overall mental illness and mental health challenge.

Leadership has evolved to best manage a range of medical conditions in the workplace. Leadership around mental illness has certainly come a long way. However, greater understanding, acceptance and integration is imperative for the future. Further evolution in workplaces will be required on this front. This will always remain a delicate balancing act around people's wellbeing and business productivity.

As a leader with a mental illness, I felt I made the right decision to return to the same place of work. This may have been the first time some people had direct exposure to an event of this nature. Statistics indicate it won't be the last. I hope my return to work helped normalise mental illness in some small way. It does impact people from all walks of life, often when it is least anticipated.

I believe that empathy is the X factor in great leadership. In terms of mental illness, greater empathy should be viewed in a positive light. This empathy needs to be more widespread. Wider than the number of people who bravely battle with mental illness.

Greater empathy should also extend to people who support others with mental illness. When I am stuck in the deepest darkest hole, with no foreseeable way out, it is soul destroying. Over the years, I have watched what my wife, family and closest friends also endure in my support. They support me when stuck in that deep dark hole, helplessly trying to convince me to keep going, pointing out all my strengths, with it often falling on deaf ears. This would be equally soul destroying at times.

I remained in the two-day-a-week role until the end of 2019 – approximately 6 months. Heraclitus, the Greek philosopher, once said, "Change is the only constant in life". Nothing can last forever and to think any differently is a fallacy of the mind. This organisation and its people will always hold fond memories for me. Without the opportunity I was afforded to return to the same workplace post hospitalisation, I wouldn't be where I am today. I hope that other organisations will follow a similar lead if any of their people are ever faced with a similar set of circumstances to mine.

Own All of It – Shadow Integration

The impediment to action advances the action. What stands in the way becomes the way.
– Marcus Aurelius

I was extremely nervous. This was a leap outside my comfort zone, not merely a jump. Was I even ready for this? Sharing my story with people individually was still a challenge but to share it loudly and proudly with a public audience … what the hell was I thinking?

The new year of 2020 had only just been welcomed. I was about to appear on *The Man That Can Project* podcast. It was an amazing opportunity, an opportunity that I would normally politely decline. My usual negative self-talk would stop me from embracing such a situation.

What if I said the wrong thing and pissed someone off?

What if people thought I was being inauthentic by seeking the limelight?

What if. What if. What if.

What if I shared my story and it helped someone else suffering?

What if I helped people who support others with mental illness?

What if I could fast track integrating my shadow?

I took a death breath. *Screw it, let's do this …*

'Welcome. Today's guest is Pete Bell. Pete is a proud father and husband. He is a heavy metal fan, cricket and boxing tragic. He also dabbles occasionally in work these days as the Director of Aurelius. Aurelius helps people to define, find and achieve their own version of success.'

And just like that my self-limiting beliefs shifted. My shadow was no longer hidden. I owned an identity with a greater purpose. And I had announced a major career pivot. There was no place left to run and hide now. I had just taken a huge step out the other side.

* * *

I always knew that my career would transition at some stage. I would seek a career that provided a greater purpose – a purpose achieved predominately through helping others. This is the reason I had commenced studying coaching at the time of admission to hospital.

Any role I settled on moving forward would need to focus on providing a balance. This would include being present both physically and mentally for my family. It would mean taking time to visit medical professionals and undertaking proactive self-work to responsibly manage my mental illness. There was so much more to consider than just earning an income for our family.

At this stage of my journey, finding this balanced work outcome was like walking the finest line. One wrong step either side and everything could fall apart. Moving the fight into the deeper rounds included finding this balanced work outcome. I needed work that provided me with a level of purpose and challenge but that did not encourage a repeat of dangerous historical patterns.

Any decision made about my future career was going to be heavily scrutinised. My support team were watching like Scotland Yard detectives, and so they should be. The last thing I wanted was to subconsciously start chasing the sun again. I had only started to build back broken trust with loved ones closest to me. I didn't want to jeopardise this in any way, shape or form.

There is a popular saying that states, "The cure can end up doing more damage than the disease". This perfectly captures the complexity of the situation I found myself in. An idle mind can act as the devil's playground. My obsessive-compulsive disorder can also develop if I am not purposefully engaged in life.

On face value, I can see that it may appear like a relatively straightforward solution: simply slow down and do nothing for a period of time. However, this would be similar to Icarus flying too close to the ocean: same outcome through different circumstances. I would end up drenched, not burnt, but still broken.

Even with the proper diagnosis in place, doing nothing was not the right outcome for my specific situation. Dwelling on the circumstances and feeling sorry for myself would never help. This would have actually been downright dangerous. I needed to ensure this didn't happen. I had to make major shifts in reframing my circumstances. My internal dialogue around the breakdown, and subsequent hospital visit, had to change. This required a shift from a negative experience to a positive opportunity. On this basis, I reframed my breakdown as being a breakthrough.

* * *

The Stoic philosopher Marcus Aurelius eludes to the fact that the obstacle is actually the way. Certain circumstances can be perceived as hindering forward movement. These circumstances and obstacles are your greatest opportunity, but you must be prepared to embrace them and confront the situation in a front on manner.

This core principle of Stoicism inspired me immensely. It drove my decision to pull forward a career pivot. It gave me much needed confidence. Marcus Aurelius provided self-belief. The belief to commence coaching as my professional career.

My breakdown could have been an obstacle to hinder my decision to coach but, when viewed as a breakthrough, it provided the catalyst. It enabled my coaching career. The day I decided to move forward and formally commit to coaching was a game changing moment. My mental illness, suppression of the shadow, and consequent breakdown were all flipped on their head. These elements were no longer obstacles hindering my growth; they provided the shining pathway forward for growth.

Coaching aligns better with the balanced life I required. It provides flexibility for our family. Most importantly, it is a profession that also supports the conscious incorporation of my shadow. It doesn't encourage further subconscious suppression; it enables me to own all of myself, to share my flaws in a proud and vulnerable manner. It reinforces this type of authentic behaviour.

People's internal dialogue reflects their subconscious view of themselves and the wider world. Such internal perceptions become apparent through people's external communication. As a coach, I needed to make vast improvements on this front. I was accountable to both myself and the people I coached. I needed to practice what I preached. This started with my self-talk around my mental illness.

No longer do I talk about my mental illness to myself as a weakness or in a negative frame of mind. It is just a small part of my life that needs to be managed responsibly – similar to how a diabetic must manage their diabetes.

No longer do I feel ashamed or embarrassed about my breakdown and hospital visit. I was blessed to have had this breakthrough experience. It finally delivered an accurate medical diagnosis. It inspired me to commence a more purposeful career path.

No longer do I feel a need to hide my shadow. I can only control my own perceptions around my mental illness. I have nothing to be afraid of by sharing this information openly with others. They will perceive it however they want; I have no control over this.

No longer do I question my ability to successfully coach people. I provide a refreshing point of difference: raw and transparent honesty around what I am and what I am not. Likewise, I have an upfront, no bullshit approach around what I can, and cannot, help people with.

The human desire to connect with what is real is summed up well by author Sue Fitzmaurice. She insinuates that people are not always interested in whether you've stood with the great. They are sometimes more interested in whether you've sat with the broken.

As a coach, I get ample practice in externally communicating my new internal dialogue. Given that the concept of the shadow can be confronting, people often ask about this part of my journey. They want to understand how the shadow integration process benefited my life.

While the benefits are wide and varied, I certainly have improved self-confidence. It has helped me become centred again and given me greater internal strength. I give minimal time and bandwidth to other people's unsolicited feedback about how I should live my life. I only take on feedback from people that form part of my support network or my closest group of friends.

People undoubtedly have the best possible intentions for providing such feedback. However, they don't understand the complexities of my mental illness. Harmless advice that comes from a genuine position of care can manifest in unintended ways. It could trigger a response that sends me hurtling towards the very welcoming warm rays of the sun again. However, it is ultimately my responsibility in how I choose to process this information if it is received. This is all I can control.

Likewise, I have greater respect for others and the way they choose to live their lives. This is a key focus area for being an effective coach. Another person's framework of the world will never be the same as mine. Therefore, I need to meet everyone at their level. I must be devoid of judgement, opinion and advice. My best life, or the evolving version of myself, will never work for anyone else.

Overall, I have far healthier relationships, both with others and myself. I have developed greater awareness of not projecting my shadow and shortcomings onto people closest to me. I accept the duality that exists in every human, myself included.

My mental energy and bandwidth have improved significantly. I am no longer drained as I don't have to participate in unproductive behaviours – behaviours which have the sole intention of protecting my shadow. Carrying around heavy protective armour is exhausting. Running away from exciting opportunities due to fear that they may expose my shadow is tiring.

Most importantly, I have become present again for my girls, both mentally and physically. This alone has been worth every minute of the often-uncomfortable process of shadow integration.

Not Everything Ages Like Fine Wine – Beliefs

Don't be satisfied with stories, how things have gone for others. Unfold your own myth.
– Rumi

There is a saying that states, "What got you here, will not get you there". This perfectly articulates my journey through the fight. It highlights the significant gap in human qualities between the start and the finish: the lost person who stepped out for round one when the bell initially rang and the person I needed to be if I was to remain standing at the conclusion of the fight.

To move the fight through the deeper rounds, one particular fallacy of the mind needed challenging. Just like the human shadow, beliefs are formed at a young age in a person's life. At a relatively young age, a person's way of making sense of the world through their belief system is typically well formed.

This belief system will influence a person's thinking, decision-making and behaviour. Most beliefs are deeply ingrained at a young age. Therefore, they are extremely difficult to change. It is, however, a fallacy of the mind to think that they cannot change.

Like many people, I had a number of beliefs that had served me well through life up until the age of 38. The ensuing existential crisis highlighted that I also had some beliefs that were self-limiting. These outdated beliefs were furthering my shadow suppression and, consequently, they needed rewiring.

I often compare my mind, and its belief system, to a computer and its programming. The initial programming in a computer delivers a high level of operational efficiency. There comes a time, however, when this programming becomes outdated. Either reprogramming or a new computer is required.

The mind doesn't have a use-by date. Not like that which exists in the context of a computer or any other form of technology, nor can the mind easily be replaced. Periodic warning signs are not received by the mind to alert the user that its belief system has become outdated or, even worse, that certain beliefs are compromising its operational efficiency. It is quite the opposite; biology makes it harder for the mind to change its belief system.

Rewiring some of my outdated beliefs needed to happen. However, it is a long process that requires hard work, time, patience and repetitive thought. It is an ongoing discipline of consciously thinking different thoughts repeatedly, at least until the creation of new neural pathways occurs.

I found solace in research undertaken by neuroscientist Eleanor Maguire. Her work provided inspiration that I could rewire my beliefs, despite the obvious challenges. Maguire identified that taxi drivers in London often have a large lump in their hippocampus. This part of the brain controls visual orientation, spatial representation and memory.

This lump was created through the overstimulation of the hippocampus. This overstimulation occurred from repetitively undertaking tasks required for their job. Muscles are strengthened and grow with the repetitive activity of lifting weights. Similarly, the mind can change and grow. This occurs through consciously thinking new thoughts.

* * *

I have undertaken a vast amount of work to rewire my own beliefs. One of the key belief focus areas was around my perception of success. The knowledge of my mental illness has played an integral role in this process. My attention has turned to the importance of leaving an appropriate legacy as success. I feel this focus has been brought forward a number of years.

My beliefs around the type of legacy I have chosen to leave have also been challenged. Financially contributing to our family is non-negotiable. I must provide for the basic cost of living, like food, shelter and education. However, the greatest gift I now believe I can leave for our family is not linked to financial benefits. It is taking full responsibility for my mental illness. This will enable the brightest future for our family.

I now have a better appreciation for a human's psychological development journey. A child's formative, middle and adolescent years are critical in this process. I must be fully present for my daughter at this foundational time of her life, both physically and mentally. It is my mental capacity and presence that is likely to generate the strongest benefit.

To provide her with the best future, I must remain balanced. I can't be riddled with obsessive thoughts and highly anxious. I can't be easily irritated, unpredictable and become disproportionately frustrated. Like my parents did so effectively with me, I must play an active role in her development. I need to have the mental bandwidth to achieve this. I want to be present to ask educators the right questions regarding her development in the future, actively monitoring her wellbeing and growth.

In terms of beliefs around my own self-worth and evolution, I have also had to rewire my frame of success. No longer does success need to follow the typical linear growth trajectory. The modern way of life, and system, reinforces that growth is a forward moving linear process. It starts as early as day care. When the first step is taken through the door, the world sets upon driving home the expectation of school being next. So commences society's 'what's next?' challenge.

This challenge frames that success is dependent upon achieving more in the future. As people age, they can come to question these societal expectations. These achievements could best be described as arbitrary from a personal perspective, especially given that they often take away the capacity to fully live in the present moment. It is a challenge to show gratitude for what is real and already in existence.

Chasing the sun is very much a forward-moving, growth trajectory pattern. Before I fell, I did get a look at the centre of the sun – as close as I am ever going to see in my lifetime anyway. It did not feel like society's systemic view of success. It felt hollow. It felt like a mindless existence.

Everyone's version of success is different. I had been following society's pathway of perceived success for too long. I should have been following my own. This all changed post my existential crisis. Once again, when framed as a breakthrough moment, it provided me with much needed inner courage. Courage to rewire outdated self-limiting beliefs. Courage to confidently dance to the beat of my own drum. Courage to pursue my own version of success.

The Fallacy of Control – Create My Certainty

The oldest, shortest words, 'yes' and 'no', are those which require the most thought.
– Pythagoras

During the fight, I had the pleasure of catching up with a mentor. This kind man had played a significant role in shaping my life, from both a personal and professional development perspective. Our conversation led to a discussion about a very challenging and uncertain period he had faced in life.

I said, "Losing your partner and having to raise multiple young children on your own must have been really tough".

The response received was something I will never forget.

He calmly replied, "It was actually the opposite. It forced me to gain clarity and find certainty. All I had to do was feed, shelter and educate my children. If something didn't align with those priorities, I simply gave it no airtime".

The timing of this conversation was serendipitous. It aligned perfectly with the reading I was regularly undertaking on Stoicism. The Stoic philosopher Epictetus once said, "First say to yourself what you would be; and then do what you have to do". On face value, this would appear alarmingly simple. The balanced life I needed also had to be rooted in simplicity.

However, simple does not always mean easy, nor does it mean non-productive or less valuable. I now have greater appreciation that the simplest things in life are often the most challenging and rewarding. The modern world has done an excellent job of over complicating itself, whether it be through technological advancements or unrealistic social expectations. The speed of life has evolved rapidly, and this is likely only to intensify in the future.

While society has evolved at a rapid rate, some functions of the human brain remain primitive, with links back to the prehistoric era. This is more than just an interesting scientific observation. My brain also contains faulty wiring. Therefore, any approach to life must respect both these facts. I needed to double down on the simplification.

Creating my own certainty and clarity was imperative. Focus solely on what I could control. This was non-negotiable. To achieve this, it was fundamental to construct the equivalent of a very strong rule book: a mental model and belief system that provided permission to say no, to put boundaries in place as required.

This was similar to most successful business strategies. The benefit comes from defining what opportunities or activities won't be pursued. Success comes from not losing sight of core business focus areas. I required a very similar style of blueprint. My self-confidence had started to improve through the centring process. However, a more proactive mechanism was still required, something that would enable me to stand strong, despite the unpredictable and messy nature of life.

Thankfully, Stoicism reintroduced me to the strength of values-based living. Once again, a relatively simple concept on face value, but I was amazed how difficult it was to initially prioritise the key core values in my life. I have developed a consistent and conscious awareness of my values. I also authentically articulate these at appropriate occasions externally. This process has enabled the certainty and clarity I required.

The power in authenticity comes from sharing your values loudly and proudly. If my behaviour does not align with the values I portray, I become incongruent. My support network, and closest group of friends, are empowered to respectfully pull me back into values alignment.

In this regard, I had a timely conversation with my psychologist. I was considering taking on greater responsibility in assisting others with mental illness. My psychologist reminded me that family was my number one priority in life. I had communicated this externally on regular occasions. Therefore, avoiding increasing my workload was more aligned behaviour. As she so eloquently put, "Just because I could do something, doesn't mean I should".

I now consciously appreciate that I will never be able to control most things in my life. I became more accepting of this irrefutable law of the universe as the fight progressed deeper. Despite this, I managed to define and create my version of certainty and clarity through only nine simple words. Simple words that are powerful. They provide me with a bullet-proof decision-making framework.

I will be the best husband and parent possible.

It's amazing how much easier the fight became once I cemented these nine words in stone. If it is not in the best interests of our family, it is not in the best interests of me.

What You Do Have – Gratitude

Wealth consists not in having great possessions, but in having few wants.
– Epictetus

During the fight, I found great comfort in examining a variety of processes and systems found in nature. These processes provided important context around my set of circumstances. They provided perspective.

I spent substantial time listening to music on my journey. One particular song was a regular on repeat and was by one of my favourite artists. It focused on the need for humans to shed their shadow – much like a snake sheds its skin, a natural process I found quite interesting to examine.

Along with their skin, snakes shed an accumulation of old parasites on their skin. These parasites hinder the snake's growth and ability to move forward. Much like a snake and its skin, I had to shed certain elements of myself to evolve during the fight. Most of what was shed was no longer productive and had to be removed.

Self-limiting beliefs were one key element that I needed to remove for good reason. However, there was another critical component of myself that was shed for different reasons. It had been removed to teach me a valuable lesson about gratitude. I certainly did not want it to be removed on a permanent basis.

The lesson I so desperately needed to learn from this process was to never take for granted the amazing gifts that already existed in my life. When I was uncontrollably chasing the sun, I sadly lost reality of all the amazing things I already had in my life. The path I was on did not encourage a level of gratitude that was commensurate with what already existed in my life.

Post the hospitalisation process, I made a decision to stop wearing my wedding ring. As I explained to my wife, I didn't stop wearing it because I no longer wanted to be married. I stopped wearing it as I felt I had lost the right to wear it. I needed to earn my wedding ring again; I needed to feel gratitude for my marriage and my family. Being the best husband and parent possible would result in a return to where it rightly belonged.

* * *

There is a wise saying around happiness: the moment it stops being heavily coveted, it will finally emerge. The concept of happiness has changed for me on my journey. The general perception, or society's consensus of what happiness may feel like, still remains somewhat relevant.

So, what does happiness look like for me now?

Happiness is a feeling that best emulates having an untroubled mind.

For obvious reasons, I often get asked now if I am happy? It is a question that really stumps me. Upon answering, I try as best as possible to avoid a thirty-minute philosophical conversation. The concept of happiness is not universal across all people. Having to explain exactly what an untroubled mind encompasses is also not straightforward. So, I simply smile and say I am balanced. Or, I am being a good husband and father. People appear to find my response relatable.

Showing gratitude undoubtedly contributes to my state of an untroubled mind. It is so important that it now forms a critical part of our family rituals. It has become a regular and disciplined practice in our household.

Every night, before dinner, our family practices gratitude. Everyone takes a turn at sharing what they were most grateful for from their day. The responses from the girls are as valuable as pieces of gold. I receive the most amazing pieces of information and insight on a daily basis.

Very rarely does a response relate to anything of material value. A show of gratitude for air-conditioning on a hot summer's day, or similar, may get mentioned occasionally. Generally, gratitude is shown for the connection and the togetherness of our family unit.

This ritual has helped me adjust to a more balanced life. It provides a real-time feedback loop that enables me to stay on the right path. I can prioritise the right things in my life. Based on the girls' feedback, I can determine if I am delivering as the best husband and parent possible.

Maintaining congruency between behaviour and values is never an easy task. Life always delivers distractions and temptations that subconsciously encourage taking a different path. It is a challenge not to take such paths when they are presented, even when it is a path that is not right to follow. Remaining authentic through living my values requires constant effort, mindfulness and conscious awareness. This is the hard work I now like to focus on because the return on investment, an untroubled mind, simply can't be matched by any material object or form of self-achievement.

Like every human, I still have days when my ego tries to get the better of me. Even little things like a newspaper article can trigger an old subconscious belief pattern. I start to ruminate on the sudden loss of my professional identity. In many ways, the only identify I once had. But then, I hear our little girl say what she was most grateful for from her day, like her dad being able to drop her off and pick her up from day care. I return quickly; I become totally grounded in the present moment again.

I still have to earn an income for our family – not just to pay the bills but also for my wellbeing and sense of purpose. Like everyone, this means I still work weekends and obscure hours occasionally. What has been interesting to observe is the girls' response to this. They show gratitude towards my work for the value it adds to our family. This would not have taken place when I was subconsciously chasing the sun. Not a single person, including myself, had any idea what I was trying to add value to.

I am sure the girls get frustrated with me at times. If I hear them wish for something new or different, I now respond subconsciously. I respectfully acknowledge the desire but follow with a key question: "What great things already exist that could satisfy this new or different desire?"

In reality, I do this more for my benefit than theirs. The repetitive questioning and behaviour help me to build the new neural pathways I require, pathways to remind me that everything that leads to a fulfilled life already exists right in front of my eyes. It is all a matter of framing this existing picture effectively, a process that is solely within my control.

The Test

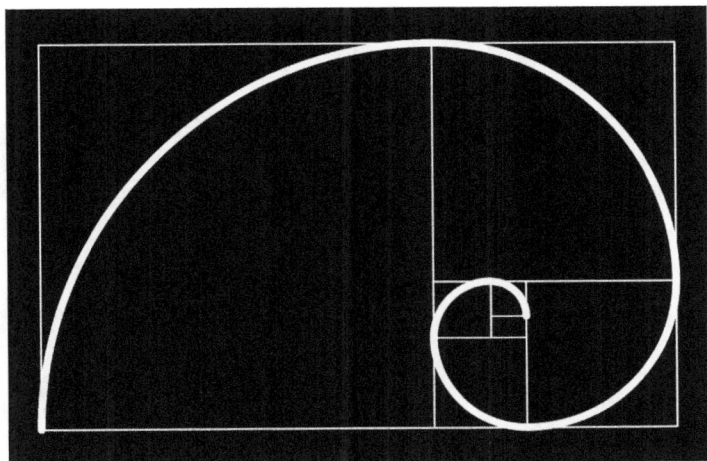

Constantly regard the universe as one living being, having one substance and one soul.

– Marcus Aurelius

On Wednesday 4th March 2020, I was excited to attend a different type of movie with my wife. It was about the life of the late philosopher Alan Watts; many of his famous lectures were shared on the big screen. We shared a quick meal of sushi before the film was due to commence. Over dinner, we joked that this was the third mid-week date night we had been on over as many weeks. It felt similar to when we were first married and free from the responsibility of parenting.

It just so happened that I had also arranged all of these date nights. This was more than I would have arranged over the previous three years. I could certainly tell my wife appreciated this improved effort and focus. Like many people early in the new year, I sensed we both felt like life had turned a corner. The year 2020 would deliver more joy, especially following a challenging 2019.

On the drive home, we were discussing some of the philosophical viewpoints from the movie. A prominent part of the conversation was around the universe ultimately being in control, how humans play a very small but still integral role in the wider universe. I insinuated that humans are wired to get ahead of themselves at times, in context of the wider system. I am sure my wife thought I was being borderline negative with some of my views. I mentioned that, if provided an inch enough times, humans will subconsciously start looking to take a mile. Put simply, humans can be driven by greed.

The human race has proven to be exceptional at adapting to change. However, something much bigger than themselves must facilitate the initial change process. They need to be shocked into action. The superior thinking capabilities of humans is both a blessing and a curse. Humans can advance their own world, the world they perceive anyway, in an impressive manner. This doesn't make them exempt from the same rule book that governs the entire universe.

* * *

The timing of this discussion was interesting to say the least. We were blissfully unaware at the time. People were just starting to purchase toilet paper in bulk; they were preparing for the looming coronavirus pandemic. We were right on the doorstep of witnessing the duality that exists in human nature: the wonderful and the not so wonderful.

It was almost one year to the day since I had left hospital. The wider system, the human race and I were about to be tested like never before. The coronavirus had arrived. This was going to be interesting. I had a history of obsessive thoughts around germs and resultant compulsive behaviour of handwashing. The bell for the final round of the fight hadn't just been rung; it exploded like a nuclear bomb blast.

The Universe Speaking

To get everything you want is not a good thing; disease makes health seem sweet, hunger leads to the appreciation of being full-fed, and tiredness creates the enjoyment of resting.
– Heraclitus

Probably like most people, I did not see the coronavirus coming, nor did it matter anyway. As I am continually learning from Stoicism, the next battle front will always be on the horizon. However, the coronavirus outbreak could be the make or break of my fight. It could manifest as a major setback to the growth and progress I had experienced over the previous year or it could further test and strengthen my resolve for the path I had now chosen.

I was quietly confident of a favourable outcome. I was reading the key principles of Stoicism proactively on a disciplined and daily basis. With this knowledge in place, I was determined not to succumb to any previous fallacies of the mind, fallacies that had contributed to my less than ideal circumstances.

The universe had spoken, I now had to make a conscious choice regarding how I would like to respond. This was the perfect set up. I was provided with a challenging test, an opportunity to put into practice all the theoretical work I had just undertaken. What could I or could I not control during this global pandemic?

* * *

I was now benefiting from the daily practice of implementing multiple Stoic principles. However, one principle in particular stood out at this specific point in time. I had become far more accepting of the fact that life simply cannot be good all the time. It is potentially the ultimate fallacy of the mind.

Nothing in nature, the world or humanity can exist on a permanent basis. This is just one of many irrefutable laws of the universe that repeats itself over and over again. As challenging as it may be to accept this, I personally find it deeply powerful and beneficial in assisting my fight to live a more balanced life.

It advances my capability for seeking an untroubled mind on a more sustainable basis. This was evident in my state of calmness through the initial phase of the coronavirus outbreak. The world was in a major state of flux. Counterintuitively, I felt in control.

This was not based on the fact that my balanced life could now minimise the full brunt of the coronavirus. I was certainly no longer as exposed as I may have been if I was still operating at the extremes and chasing the sun. However, our family's life, just like everyone else's, was still impacted in a less than favourable manner by the outbreak.

The Stoic philosopher Seneca provides a shining light on this front during his reflections after the burning down of the colony of Lyons. Seneca indicates that the fire, and subsequent destruction, was a terrible situation. No person wanted this to happen, nor could they have predicted its occurrence. However, he noted that, through examining nature, a level of comfort could still be derived from the sad state of events. Historically, the significant in stature have fallen on multiple occasions. Through a transformative process, they have equally emerged out the other side in a better position. This time-tested wisdom of Stoic philosophers, like Seneca, helped guide my decision; my choice around how I would answer the calling of the coronavirus was clear cut. I set about determining only the elements I could control. I applied a laser-like focus to execute these tasks. Anything that existed outside of my control received zero bandwidth. The resultant isolation associated with coronavirus also provided opportunity. I could rekindle my passion for lost creative endeavours. I started playing the drums again and writing.

This story may never have been documented without the coronavirus – or the Stoics, who ensured I made the most of this unforeseen, and interesting, period of time. It was not lost on me that Marcus Aurelius wrote down his ideas, that went on to become Meditations, during the Antonine Plague. This historical moment of brilliance alone provided ample inspiration.

The coronavirus will come and go. The universe, at some point in the future, will speak again, just to remind everyone of who is ultimately in control. Stoicism has taught me the ability to reframe life's predictably unpredictable events. So, whatever the universe delivers in the future, I have a mind that is better prepared to view it from a different perspective: a wiser prescriptive, a philosophical viewpoint, an overall better perspective.

Good Enough for Marcus; Good Enough For Me

The tranquillity that comes when you stop caring what they say. Or think, or do. Only what you do.
– Marcus Aurelius

During the fight, I put so much self-work and effort into building my internal strength and courage. I had to learn, and practice, that my wellbeing and state of an untroubled mind can ultimately only be determined by me. Other people's behaviour, emotions and views were outside of my control. Therefore, they could not play such a dominant role in determining my self-value, emotional state, or overall perspective on life.

In light of the coronavirus challenge, on two specific occasions, my emotions did get the better of me. My emotions were driven by comments made directly from others.

Our little girl had only just turned three years old when I was admitted to hospital. It played on my mind for a period of time whether she would remember this experience in the future. However, everyone I had spoken with about the matter eased my concerns. They confirmed that she would probably have been too young to remember much, if anything.

I was putting her to bed one night in late March 2020, when she cuddled up to my leg with her pink rug in hand. I was a little flustered, as bedtime is not always a straightforward task. At first, I wasn't sure if I had heard her question correctly.

Looking up at me, she asked, "Daddy, do you remember the happy meal and the lollies I had when we came to see you in hospital?"

I responded with "Pardon?"

"You know, that time you were in hospital and couldn't be at home".

"Well yes. I do remember," I said.

"Please don't ever go back to hospital, Daddy. I missed you too much and Mumma and I need you here with us at home."

"I won't leave ever again," I said, with tears welling up in my eyes.

We hugged tightly before starting the bed tuck-in process.

A few days later, my wife and I were sharing a conversation with a close friend. This friend was aware of the challenging period of time that we had just worked through. They asked, from a position of care, how we were coping since the coronavirus outbreak.

Before I could answer, my wife jumped in and confidently said, "We are going really well, thanks. Pete has already calmly taken control of what is required for our family to ensure we get through as best as possible.

I could not think of a better partner to have by my side during this tough period". I cannot put words on paper just yet to explain what this meant to me.

At that given moment, a large proportion of any remaining guilt I had was lifted straight from my shoulders. It finally hit home to me just how far I had come in terms of rebuilding the trust that had deteriorated – a deterioration that had occurred on my watch.

These two events, that took place in close succession with the girls, was enough evidence to signify to me that I had closed out the current fight. I had become a highly valued, balanced and contributing member of our family once again.

It was undoubtedly a joyous feeling that resulted from this positive reinforcement. However, as equally as important, I internally believed that I was headed down the right path. Despite the world being turned upside down from the coronavirus, the existence of my untroubled mind had led me to believe this. I felt very centred.

Before these two events, I had also begun to wear my wedding ring again. No one else's views factored into this decision. It was a symbol to me that I was ready again. I had earned the right as a husband and parent. Overall, I felt amazing.

There is often a view that Stoicism totally discourages any emotion. Rightly or wrongly, my interpretation of the philosophy is that emotion remains a critical component of a healthy existence. However, like all elements of life, it must remain balanced and within the right context.

In my opinion, the ultimate Stoic role model was Marcus Aurelius. I firmly believe him to be the Greatest of All Time, or as per the modern vernacular, the G.O.A.T. Marcus Aurelius showed emotion; he was human. Marcus even cried. The man endured significant loss and hardship, including the passing of eight children. How could a healthy, well-balanced human not show emotion in such situations?

I experienced numerous emotional, but equally rewarding, moments during the coronavirus pandemic. Documenting this story in itself was a highly emotive experience at times. These were touching, human moments. They were moments that I must never forget.

The Second Half

Life can only be understood backwards, but it must be lived forwards.
– Soren Kierkegaard

So, I made it through to the twelfth round still standing. I would love to say that we had a massive celebration to mark such an achievement, but this would have been irresponsible behaviour on my behalf.

The speed of my fight is no doubt the perceived elephant in the room, even for me. Getting back up off the canvas to fight again is like riding a bike. I have had so much practice, yet even I was caught by surprise this time.

My support team is well aware of this. I am now monitored like a hawk, something for which I am extremely grateful. At times, they questioned the sometimes-intense process of putting this story on paper. This was the right course of action, but I needed to prove it was a balanced exercise. While it is great to help others, it can't be at the cost of myself or our family.

Academic research published in the July 2016 edition of the scientific journal *Molecular Psychiatry* found that obsessive-compulsive disorder sufferers are ten times more likely to commit suicide than the general population. I must never forget this. While confronting, this is life-changing knowledge. On this basis, I won't ever put a finite completion date on my recovery. This could lull me back into a false sense of security.

* * *

I have since revisited the work of psychologist Carl Jung with new-found intrigue. He often described life as having two distinct halves. His thinking resonates strongly on this front, given my journey.

According to Jung, the first half of life typically lasts for between 36 to 40 years. For some people, this can take longer. This first half of life is full of expansion into the world. It is about building the ego, creating an external identity, feeling important, taking on the world. At the hands of failure or significant loss, middle life produces a noted shift. People come to realise that the conscious self is not all of them; it is merely what is acceptable to them.

In the second half of life, people usually become more reflective. A real purpose and identity are sought at a deeper level, far deeper than the external-facing identity and image people fight so hard to protect during the first half of their life. No longer is any strong meaning found in being successful, especially as it relates to material items or society's 'what's next?' pressure and challenge. People find their true self and inner identity.

* * *

There is one part of this story that I grappled with most in relation to whether I should, or should not, share it. It is still raw in many ways. It is also still real and something I battle with in my own mind: the stigma surrounding mental illness.

This stigma has improved. Despite this, my personal experience is that there is still a way to travel. The conscious words people use often give away their subconscious beliefs. People don't always realise this; it happens outside of their conscious control. As a coach, I am tuned in to identify these nuances. I sometimes witness this when sharing my story.

The majority of people wholeheartedly support my journey. Their conscious and subconscious responses are congruent. A smaller number of people want to support my journey but, at a subconscious level, I can identify that their belief system won't enable this.

Their subconscious still believes that mental illness is a sign of weakness. This manifests through non-direct, or non-deliberate, insinuations including:

- That my resilience is questionable.
- That my hospitalisation was avoidable or that others endure similar hardship but never have to go to hospital.
- That what I did was admirable but is not a path that others would ever consider going down, given their superior mental strength, or that they can't be afforded such a luxury.
- That I should simply do nothing for an extended period of time, then all my problems will disappear.

Why is this important to include? Because this is exactly what I once believed.

I was a lucky one. I am so blessed that my support network took control. Otherwise, society's next sad and silent statistic would likely have been me.

Deeper, fundamental belief systems need to change around mental illness. This will benefit from time, shifts in generational viewpoints and concerted effort.

* * *

I am proud to say that my mind is currently in an untroubled state. I have worked hard to view the world with greater optimism, and this includes accepting reality – the reality that an ongoing untroubled state of mind will require a lifelong commitment of responsibility.

What does this responsibility entail?

- I must continue to accept my mental illness and integrate it fully into my life.
- I must continue to take the appropriate dosage of medication consistently.
- I must consistently check in with my support network of medical professionals, especially at full health, so they can see through my subconscious patterns if they suddenly manifest again.
- I must continue my self-work; this will be a never-ending journey of self-acceptance and care.
- I must live a values-based, balanced life; my behaviour must remain congruent with my core value set.
- I must enjoy the present moment, smiling with comfort that whatever may eventuate next is outside of my control.

- I must continue to be the best husband and parent possible.

If ever you have an opportunity to support, encourage or talk to a person suffering with a mental illness, please try your hardest to avoid the silence path. This silence is deafening on the other side of the fence. In my experience, silence hurts far greater than making an effort to say something, even if that something may not be textbook perfect.

It can be as simple as, "I am thinking of you. But I want to give you space until you are ready. Take your time and please let me know when you are ready. I will be here for you".

I received a multitude of these types of messages when I was unwell. I will never forget those messages, nor the kind-hearted souls who sent them to me or my wife. Those few words do have the potential to save a person's life. That has to be worth the potential uncomfortable feeling of sending them in the first place.

In closing ... I sincerely hope reading this book has provided value to you. Even if it is:

- Just the smallest glimmer of hope.
- Encouragement to wait and see what the universe may have in store next.
- A spark to keep moving forward on the journey.
- Self-belief to take another small, but important, step – a step that could lead, compound and grow.
- Stepping out the other side into the future.

May the gentle warmth from the sun just touch the top of your wings. May the temperate ocean coolness softly skim the underside of your chest. May you find the inner strength to be at peace with yourself and the universe, whatever comes your way.

– Pete Bell

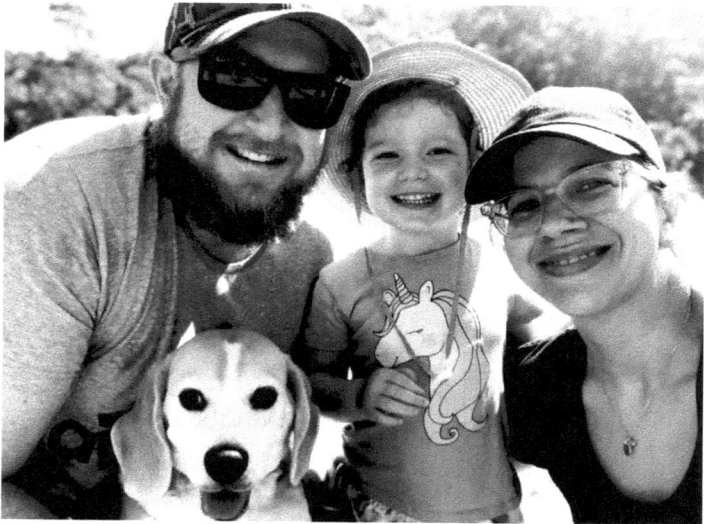

A Partner's Perspective

Stretching their hand up to reach the stars, too often people forget the flowers at their feet.
— Jeremy Bentham

When Pete told me he was going to document and publish his journey, I wasn't surprised. He had been through a life-changing experience with valuable learnings about mental illness, resilience and courage. He was now committed to helping people where possible and, if his story could make a difference to just one person, it would be worth it. And, well, the world had plunged into a global pandemic, which meant a lot more time at home, so why not?

What did surprise me is that I felt that I also wanted to contribute.

I'm not an author, nor an expert on mental illness or self-discovery. What I can offer, however, is another perspective: a very important perspective. As conveyed throughout the story, stepping out the other side relies on a team of committed people. Fighting such battles alone is otherwise – no doubt – harrowing and, sadly, may not have the same positive outcome.

I feel I can offer some useful insights for relatives, friends and colleagues. Information that may assist you in supporting others in the future. Pete uses the analogy of a boxing fight for his story. I liken my story to being in the trenches alongside someone. When you choose to dive into the trenches alongside someone you love or someone in need, the lessons learned are equally valid and valuable.

* * *

Like Pete, I did not see that Tuesday hospital admission coming, nor did I think he had an undiagnosed mental illness. We had always just believed that he suffered from some general mental health challenges, like all humans do.

Only 24 hours earlier, I went to the office for a normal work day with an expectation to commute home, have dinner with the family and do it all again the next day. It was working parent life and, not long after a rare four-week break over Christmas, I'm pretty sure I was already thinking about our Easter holiday plans.

While I was focused on the future, my irritatingly intelligent, funny and hard-working husband had been falling into a completely frightening standstill. One quick conversation with Pete was all it took; I knew this was not a normal set of circumstances. What might have appeared sudden on the outside was probably a long and extended period of pain and suffering on the inside.

When my husband rang that morning and franticly said he needed to see a doctor immediately, I dropped everything and went straight home to see him. My decision to attend the doctor's appointment with him that day was critical in hindsight. With multiple caring eyes on him, Pete finally found the courage to open up about how low he really was. I had seen him low before but never previously at the depths of this new and scary level.

I remember feeling very grateful and relieved that the medical professional also witnessed what I did that day. We benefited from their years of vast medical experience. They made the right judgement call with Pete. Like any situation, expert advice and knowledge are absolutely essential in decision-making. We were to make many more big decisions in the months following this initial doctor's appointment.

* * *

The obsessive-compulsive disorder diagnosis provided me with relief, but also frustration and uncertainty. Some people informed me that it could take two years before a level of stability in our lives returned. We had been given a rope out of the trenches, but it was still deep, muddy and a long climb. How had this information been unknown for so long and what exactly did it mean for our future?

Still, a proper diagnosis was powerful knowledge and Pete could now start climbing if he wanted to. But I had to climb too, and I'm sure my commitment helped him to get up the rope faster. He knew we would climb together.

Looking back now, and thinking about Pete's obvious inner conversations, often breaks my heart. Seemingly overnight, he was often at war with himself and decided to punish himself at every opportunity. He also gave everything to certain things (the compulsions) and nothing to others. To someone close, and if unexplained, this behaviour can appear selfish and provide a solid roadblock to relying on that person consistently.

Therefore, before anything else, I had to learn more about obsessive-compulsive disorder, anxiety and how to live with it because you simply cannot fix it. And what if our daughter experiences something like this one day?

I attended appointments, asked the doctors multiple questions, read the fact sheets and reviewed the online resources (tip: avoid the Google rabbit hole). I read the articles Pete would send me (and still does). I mapped out the required treatment commitments every week, where Pete needed to be and how this would fit into our usual schedule. Supporting him to be independent and to take responsibility for his part in the climb was strongly advised, and I saw obvious benefits.

I needed help too. I visited a psychologist and attended an obsessive-compulsive disorder support group for partners. I empathised with the potential life-destroying impact this illness could have and, consequently, resolved to play my part for our family.

The financial impact can be real. I imagine each situation is very different as there is a lot to think about: income, expenses, insurances, future job prospects. With advice, I decided to dial up my income and adjust the household budget. There was generosity offered by those around us. And it wasn't the first time, but my husband's relentless focus on savings provided peace of mind and would eventually enable a future career shift for him – a key part of the story.

I kept the inner support circle small. While I appreciated outreach from those that cared, I engaged with only who I needed to, leaned on close relatives, a colleague and maybe two friends. We had to be brave and uncomfortably honest at times. Most people find it easier to ask about the partner's progress. Pete and I often discussed what and how to share information and who we shared it with. In the early weeks, I had to take the lead on some of these uncomfortable discussions.

A small support circle is useful because managing your own mental health, supporting someone else and generally getting your family's future back on track is hard work, confronting and tiring. Further to this, not everyone around you will relate or empathise. But that is ok. As you're climbing out of the trenches, there is no energy to manage more than your immediate priorities like children, pets, work and a handful of expectations. There's definitely nothing available for anyone who isn't giving you what you need. To this extent, I was hesitant to take on big professional or personal projects until the time was right.

* * *

There were slips during the climb out of the trenches. I felt huge anxiety about leaving Pete alone more than once. I didn't know all the right things to say or do, or if I was being a good partner. I grieved for the familiarity of our former life, the partner I wanted and the co-parent I needed.

Much later, Pete likened the events to a kind of accident, and the resulting 'brain' injury had led to an important diagnosis. The breakdown became a breakthrough. As I had experienced since we first met, despite all of his inner turmoil, Pete's insights would again be truly enlightening and further strengthen my admiration for him.

As covered in this book, we've made our way out of the trenches and are enjoying life again. First, we have our health and each other. That's definitely worth celebrating. Next, there is a renewed sense of purpose that we will forever be better placed to help others. Supporting Pete in a pathway that directly helps other people, and himself, is incredibly rewarding. Lastly, our family is more connected and present – nothing like a breakthrough experience to sharpen your focus on family values and what really matters.

For me, stepping out the other side was just as important. It provided a much-needed nudge in a better direction for our family. I am under no illusions; life will deliver us new trenches in the future. However, we will fight out of these with greater experience, resilience and, thanks to Pete, a whole lot of ancient wisdom to turn to.

Rhianne Bell

May 2020

Next Steps

A number of the non-medical learnings that have been documented in this story have been incorporated into a specific coaching program that may assist others. This coaching program is delivered by Pete Bell through a platform known as Aurelius. Aurelius is focused on adding maximum value to people and business below the surface so that they can shine above it.

As conveyed in this book, the best version of a person already exists deep within themselves. Often, the facilitation of a process founded in mutual trust can help bring these distinctive human qualities to the surface. This process requires a balanced approach that typically combines learned experience, humility, openness, transparency and vulnerability.

The strategies and frameworks applied by Aurelius also have links back to philosophies that have stood the test of time, such as Stoicism. They are rooted in the principle that only one person can ultimately be responsible for defining, finding and living their own version of success. Unfortunately, there is no silver bullet or clearly defined formula in this regard, but a trusted partner can assist on this journey.

Life is messy, and success can be equally as messy.

Aurelius is passionate about supporting community initiatives, including breaking down the stigma associated with mental illness, improving the dialogue around suicide and providing shelter for the disadvantaged.

For further information on the Aurelius coaching program, please visit:

Aurelius

www.aurelius.com.au

Mental Health Support Services

As covered in the Author's Note at the start of this story, please seek appropriate help immediately for any personal suffering. A list of important support services is detailed below.

Beyondblue Support Service
Phone: 1300 22 4636
www.beyondblue.org.au/get-support/get-immediate-support

Headspace
Phone: 1800 650 890
http://www.headspace.org.au/

Kids Help Line
Phone: 1800 55 18 00
http://www.kidshelp.com.au/

Lifeline
Phone: 13 11 14
http://www.lifeline.org.au/

Mensline Australia
Phone: 1300 78 99 78
http://www.mensline.org.au/

ReachOut.com
http://au.reachout.com/

SANE Australia
Phone: 1800 187 263
http://www.sane.org/index.php

Suicide Call Back Service
Phone: 1300 659 467
https://www.suicidecallbackservice.org.au/

List of Resources

A number of valuable information sources contributed to this story. The organisations that contain these important people; plus films and other resources are listed below.

The Practical Stoic Podcast
https://www.simonjedrew.com/practicalstoicpodcast/

Poker Face – Men's Mental Health
https://www.facebook.com/saveitforthetable/

The Man That Can Project
https://www.themanthatcanproject.com/

The Eighth Mile Consulting
https://eighthmile.com.au/

Suicide Prevention Pathways
https://suicidepreventionpathways.org.au/

Orygen - Youth Mental Health - Helping young Australians
https://www.orygen.org.au/

CEOsage Shadow Training
https://scottjeffrey.com/shadow-course/

Why Not Now! Alan Watts
https://www.youtube.com/watch?v=tW8XSlgTDd8

Acknowledgements

Rhianne, a modern-day Stoic. Thank you for supporting me to share this story and contributing in such a valuable manner.

Family and closest friends. Thank you for your unconditional support, not just for me, but also for the girls. You never falter.

My medical support team. Thank you for taking the time to work with me and being courageous enough to challenge the status quo. While our journey has only started together, I am confident and ready for whatever comes next with you consistently in my corner.

My past work colleagues. Thank you for your care and support. This would not have been an easy task. I wouldn't be where I am today without your welcoming arms that enabled me back into the workplace. To Brook and others, your ongoing commitment to stay in touch, despite my now different journey, makes you true friends.

My current work colleagues. Thank you for the friendship, support and belief. You inspire me daily and remind me how important it is to stay true to the real self. It is a pleasure to stand beside you all.

Simon from *The Practical Stoic Podcast*. Thank you for the amazing foreword, guidance and wisdom. You help me to see the world with a much clearer lens. I am excited about your big future and look forward to watching your journey continue as a friend. Never stop doing what you do.

Professor Patrick McGorry from *Oyrgen*. Thank you for taking the time to read my story and provide such kind words of support. I am still pinching myself that a person of your high calibre, who has made such a prolific positive impact in the mental health space, afforded me your valuable time and support. My words can't do justice to exactly what this means to me.

Peter, Richard and the team at *Suicide Prevention Pathways*. Thank you for supporting me with this story, and partnering to ensure the message assists as many people as possible. I am really looking forward to working closely with you in the future and supporting your extremely important work.

Chris at *Poker Face*, Lachie at *The Man That Can Project* and Dave at *The Eighth Mile Consulting*. Thank you for believing in my new journey and providing support. Never underestimate the positive influence you have on the lives of so many people. Never stop doing what you do.

My dedicated proofreaders. Your commitment and attention to detail was phenomenal. Thank you also for believing in me to continue on the path to share this story, especially when the self-doubt kicked in.

The team at Brisbane Self Publishing Service. Thank you for helping me bring this story to life. It never would have happened without your expertise, support and profession-alism.

.

About the Author

Peter Bell is the owner of Aurelius, a management consulting firm which focuses on adding maximum value to businesses and people below the surface so that they can shine above it. His people, strategy and research skills have been honed over more than 20 years of experience within diverse roles and sectors.

He is passionate about breaking down the stigma associated with mental illness and bringing the subject of suicide out into the open.

Peter lives in Brisbane, Queensland with his wife and daughter who are his everything.

www.ingramcontent.com/pod-product-compliance
Lightning Source LLC
Chambersburg PA
CBHW071418210326
41597CB00020B/3567